The Prescription Drug Guide for Nurses

The Prescription Drug Guide for Nurses

Sue Jordan

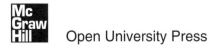

Open University Press

Open University Press
McGraw-Hill Education
McGraw-Hill House
Shoppenhangers Road
Maidenhead
Berkshire
England
SL6 2QL

email: enquiries@openup.co.uk
world wide web: www.openup.co.uk

and Two Penn Plaza, New York, NY 10121-2289, USA

First published 2008

A catalogue record of this book is available from the British Library

ISBN-13: 978-0-33-522547-7 (pb)   978-0-33-522546-0 (hb)
ISBN-10: 0-33-522547-0 (pb)   0-33-522546-2 (hb)
Library of Congress Cataloging-in-Publication Data
CIP data applied for

Typeset by RefineCatch Limited, Bungay, Suffolk
Printed in Great Britain by Bell & Bain Ltd, Glasgow

The McGraw·Hill Companies

Dedication: my family

Acknowledgements

Laura Downes, special projects manager *RCN Publishing*, Gwen Clarke, Art and Science editor *Nursing Standard*. Tim Madge, managing editor new media, *RCN Publishing*, for inspiration and support. Professor Melanie Jasper, Professor Gareth Morgan, Swansea University, Rachel Crookes, Jack Fray and James Bishop, Open University Press, for help and support. Jeffrey Aronson, editor of *Meyler's Side Effects of Drugs*, for such a wonderful resource. Stephen Storey, librarian, School of Health Sciences, Swansea University, for tireless assistance. Peter Gardiner, medical illustrator, Clinical Skills Ltd.

Contents

vii

Preface

Prescription drugs: theory to practice

This book applies pharmacology to nursing practice, with the overall aim of enhancing patient care. The main focus of the book is adverse drug reactions, and the implications for patient monitoring. Adverse drug reactions account for around 4% of UK hospital admissions. Over 70% of these problems are avoidable (Pirmohamed *et al*. 2004): the monitoring of prescribed medications has long been a cause for concern (Royal College of General Practitioners 1985, DH 2000, Audit Commission 2001, Committee of Public Accounts 2006). Regular, structured patient monitoring for adverse events, as outlined in our 'Implications for Practice' charts, has the potential to reduce the incidence and severity of these problems. However, this work lies on the inter-professional boundaries between doctors, pharmacists and nurses, and might become marginalised. As with other 'boundary work', responsibilities are not clearly allocated (Jordan 2002a, 2007). Consequently, potential adverse drug reactions are not always monitored in routine care. By developing the *Nursing Standard Prescription Drug Series*, we aim to offer practical nursing strategies to minimise the ill-health caused by adverse drug reactions.

Informed patient monitoring

Drug administration is one of the highest risk activities for nurses (Gladstone 1995). Any failure to consider the details of adverse reactions, drug interactions or administration schedules may compromise the efficacy of therapeutic regimens and even patient safety. Also, nurses' professional status may be compromised if they fail to ensure that the highest standards of drug administration are observed. By considering the pedagogic interpretation of nursing pharmacology, and offering practical suggestions, this book aims to help professionals reduce the number and severity of adverse drug reactions. It thereby aims to contribute to public and professional protection.

Evidence-based practice: the state of the evidence

Ideally, every practice activity would be based on the results of randomised, multiple blind, parallel group, placebo controlled pragmatic clinical trials of adequate size, supported by large cohort studies and service users' views. While these standards are sometimes achieved by those investigating the benefits of drugs, there has been no comparable investment in research into the adverse effects of medications. There is even less research funding available to explore strategies to monitor and minimise adverse drug reactions. Therefore, suggestions for practice are proffered from a theoretical, rather than a statistical, standpoint. Nevertheless, we hope that patients and practitioners will find them helpful in their day to day lives and practice.

Professor Jane Robinson FRCN, MA, PhD, MCIPD, RN, RHV, HVT, ONC, Editor, *International Nursing Review* and Emeritus Professor University of Nottingham

Sue Jordan MB BCh, PhD, PGCE (FE), FHEA, Senior Lecturer, School of Health Science, Swansea University

September 2007

Using this Book

The unique feature of this book is the practice guides for the administration and patient monitoring of commonly administered prescription drugs. Patient monitoring focuses on adverse drug reactions; these are defined and classified in the introductory chapter. The 20 chapters on the most commonly administered drug groups form the core of the book. Each chapter details drug actions, indications, administration, adverse effects and practice suggestions for monitoring and ameliorating adverse effects, followed by summaries of cautions/contra-indications and interactions. Initiation of some therapeutic regimens, such as anti-cancer drugs, anti-epileptics, antipsychotics, is usually undertaken by specialists. In other areas of practice, such as symptom control or where medication is prescribed 'as needed', nurses may be more involved in decision-making, and, consequently, this book offers rather more detail on indications. However, nurses are always advised to consult specialist literature.

Many drugs can cause problems on withdrawal, and all can give rise to hypersensitivity or allergic responses, which are discussed collectively in the final section. There can be no guarantee that a prescribed medication will achieve its desired effect, and we ask practitioners to consider 'therapeutic failure'. For consistency, these topics have been placed at the end of the practice guides.

Selecting the 20 most commonly prescribed drug groups was not easy. Some drugs included are available without prescription, but are commonly prescribed in many healthcare settings. We are concerned here with the use of these medicines under supervision of healthcare professionals, rather than occasional purchases.

Information presented here is only a summary and a guide, and an outline of principles. Lists are not exhaustive. Practitioners should consult more detailed information sources, such as the *British National Formulary* on bnf.org.uk or manufacturers' data sheets on medicines.org.uk, and the secondary sources referred to in the text. The order of the chapters follows the *British National Formulary* (BNF).

Adrenaline/epinephrine: 'adrenaline' is used, to be consistent with the BNF.

Abbreviations Used in the Text

ACE	Angiotensin converting enzyme
ANS	Autonomic nervous system
BNF	*British National Formulary*
BP	Blood pressure
bpm	Beats per minute
CNS	Central nervous system
COPD	Chronic obstructive pulmonary disease
DNA	Deoxyribosenucleic acid
ECF	Extracellular fluid
FBC	Full blood count
GABA	Gamma amino butyric acid (an inhibitory neurotransmitter)
GFR	Glomerular filtration rate
GI	Gastrointestinal
H_2RA	Histamine receptor antagonist
kPa	Kilo Pascals – the SI unit of pressure
l	Litre
LFT	Liver function test
MI	Myocardial Infarction
mmHg	Millimetre of mercury, unit of pressure
NICE	National Institute of Health and Clinical Excellence
NSAID	Non-steroidal anti-inflammatory drug
PPI	Proton pump inhibitor
PSNS	Parasympathetic nervous system
RBC	Red blood cell
SNS	Sympathetic nervous system
SSRIs	Selective serotonin re-uptake inhibitors, a group of anti-depressant drugs, including fluoxetine (Prozac®)
TFTs	Thyroid function tests
WHO	World Health Organisation

List of Contributors

Mo Afzal BSc (Hons), RMN, MSc (Econ), PGCE (FE). MBA Learning and Development Manager, Substance Misuse Services, Birmingham and Solihull Mental Health Trust

David Gallimore BSc, MSc, RGN. Tutor in Adult Nursing at the School of Health Sciences, University of Wales, Swansea

Howard Griffiths RN, BSc, MSc, PGCE (FE), RNT. Clinical Practice Tutor, School of Health Sciences, Swansea University

Jeanette Hewitt RMN, RGN, RNT, BSc (Hons), PGCE, PGCertCouns. Lecturer, School of Health Sciences, Swansea University

Janet Jones RN, MSc, BEd, RNT. Lecturer in Cancer Nursing (retired), School of Health Sciences, Swansea University

John Knight BSc, PhD. Lecturer, School of Health Sciences, Swansea University

Richard Lake RN, Dip.N, BSc (Hons), ATNC. Clinical Skills Tutor, School of Health Sciences, Swansea University

Dave Pointon MA, RMN, RNT. Head of Centre for Mental Health Studies (retired), School of Health Sciences, Swansea University

Professor Jane Robinson FRCN, MA, PhD, MCIPD, RN, RHV, HVT, ONC. Editor, *International Nursing Review* and Emeritus Professor University of Nottingham

Introduction

Adverse drug reactions: definitions and classifications

While helping patients cope with the burden of illness, healthcare professionals may, some-times, overlook the burden of treatment, including adverse drug reactions. These account for around 4% of hospital admissions, and over 70% are avoidable (Pirmohamed *et al.* 2004). While medical pharmacology focuses on cure and prescribing, nursing pharmacology centres on care and monitoring. Prescribed medicines bring many benefits, but they are inevitably associated with adverse effects. These are a nursing concern. Regular, structured patient monitoring for adverse drug reactions, coupled with appropriate follow through, has the potential to reduce the numbers of people hospitalised. There are several types of adverse drug reactions and some definitions are offered here to underpin understanding and recognition of potential problems.

Definitions

Therapeutics is the treatment of disease. **Pharmacology** is the science dealing with the interactions between a living system and chemicals introduced from outside the system. A drug may be defined as any small molecule that, when introduced into the body, alters body function by interactions at molecular level.

An **adverse event** is any untoward medical occurrence in a patient or participant in a drug trial to whom a medicinal product has been administered, including occurrences which are not necessarily caused by or related to that product (ICH 1996). Distinguishing an adverse reaction to treatment from an adverse event involves assigning a cause (known as attribution of causality). Adverse events may not be attributable to treatments or drugs: for example, 89% (116/130) of healthy medical students, taking no medication, reported adverse events, most commonly headache, fatigue and nasal congestion (Meyer *et al.* 1996).

An **adverse drug reaction** (ADR) is defined as any untoward and unintended response in a patient or investigational subject to a medicinal product which is related to any dose administered (ICH 1996). A more precise definition is: 'An appreciably harmful or unpleasant reaction, resulting from an intervention related to the use of a medicinal product, which predicts hazard from future administration and warrants prevention or specific treatment, or alteration of the dosage regimen, or withdrawal of the product' (Edwards & Aronson 2000 p. 1255).

Sometimes, the adverse effects of treatment are dramatic and attribution is unequivocal, for example when six healthy volunteers became seriously ill within hours of receiving the experimental drug TGN1412 (Suntharalingam *et al.* 2006). However, adverse effects are often mundane or indistinguishable from commonplace problems (Millar 2001, Tierney 2003). For example, in a systematic review of six clinical trials, blurred vision was reported by 10/529 patients prescribed chlorpromazine and 9/381 taking placebo, a statistically non-significant difference (Adams *et al.* 2005), indicating that the cause of the blurred vision was uncertain. For some ADRs, there is insufficient research to link an adverse event with a prescription drug (Talbot & Stephens 2004). For example, patients taking statins, such as simvastatin, may experience joint stiffness or arthralgia, but identifying the cause of these common conditions can be difficult, and only careful investigation revealed the link between shoulder stiffness and statin therapy in women (Harada *et al.* 2001). More complex is the situation where adverse events may be confused with the illness being treated. For example, SSRIs are prescribed for depression and anxiety, but anxiety is a reported adverse effect of these drugs (Doran 2003, BNF 2007). Patients do not always recognise symptoms as being drug-related or report medication-related symptoms to their doctors, particularly mundane events, such as incontinence and headaches (Weingart *et al.* 2005).

Serious adverse events or reactions are defined as untoward medical occurrences that at any dose: result in death, are life-threatening, require hospitalisation or prolong hospitalisation, result in persistent or significant disability or incapacity or are congenital anomalies (ICH 1996).

Classifications: types of ADR

Adverse drug reactions (ADR) can be broadly divided into those which are dose-related (glossary) and predictable, and those which are neither. Some authorities (Edwards & Aronson 2000) include withdrawal reactions and therapeutic failure as ADRs. It may be appropriate to consider the effects of drugs administered in pregnancy and labour in a separate category, as transgenerational adverse effects. In summary ADRs are classed as:

◆ Dose-dependent or 'augmented' (type A)

◆ Unrelated to dose, unexpected, idiosyncratic or 'bizarre' (type B)

◆ Withdrawal

◆ Therapeutic failure

◆ Transgenerational effects

Dose-dependent: Most (about 75%) adverse drug reactions are dose related, for example bleeding due to unmonitored warfarin and hypoglycaemia from poorly monitored insulin were the most common adverse drug reactions responsible for hospital admission in an American study (Budnitz *et al.* 2006). These problems are more likely to arise at high doses or with overdosing (intentionally or unintentionally). Administration of interacting drugs or foods could also precipitate these problems (see warfarin). For some adverse effects, such as carcinogenicity and genetic damage, it is not always known whether the effects are dose-related (Box 1). Dose-dependent ADRs can be subdivided into:

1. **Primary effects,** relating directly to the main action of the drug, such as bleeding from excessive warfarin. These effects are entirely predictable, and patients are always closely monitored, for example, patients taking warfarin have blood clotting checked at least every 3 months.

2. **Secondary effects,** relating to incidental actions of the drug, for example, many antibiotics cause diarrhoea, and many anti-cancer drugs cause vomiting. Secondary effects may limit the dose that can be administered, which is a particular concern when working with patients with cancer. Secondary adverse effects arise because many drugs act by more than one mechanism or affect several systems of the body.

Patients at risk of dose-dependent adverse effects: Professionals should be vigilant
for adverse drug reactions in vulnerable patients, particularly those who are unable to eliminate drugs efficiently, often the very old and the very young. Women are at greater risk of adverse drug reactions than men. This may be due to differences in body composition (women have less muscle mass, reduced kidney function) or hormone balance (Routledge 2004).

Less predictably, some people may be unduly sensitive to adverse effects due to variations in their genetic make-up. Patients with reduced liver or kidney function may be unable to eliminate their medication at a normal rate. Therefore, even when given normal doses, their medication will accumulate, and may reach toxic concentrations, causing adverse effects.

Some liver enzymes (glossary) needed for drug metabolism are not functional in people with certain genetic variations. People only become aware of this situation when they are prescribed certain medication, and unexpectedly suffer severe adverse effects at relatively low doses. For example, it is estimated that 7% of Caucasians are poor metabolisers of codeine, haloperidol, several anti-depressants (including paroxetine and imipramine), and other drugs. This is caused by a defect on chromosome 22, which results in absence of a key enzyme responsible for processing these drugs (CYP2D6 in cytochrome P450) (Routledge 2004).

Box 1   Genotoxicity and carcinogenicity

The carcinogenic potential of some drugs, such as tobacco, is well known. However, the link between cancer risk and dose of carcinogen is not always known, and may not be directly tested in humans. Manufacturers test compounds in bacteria, mammalian cells and rodents to observe any changes to DNA and growth of tumours over at least 2 years (Snodin 2004). However, the results of these studies cannot necessarily be transferred to humans. Observation studies and databases indicate that the risk of lung cancer is proportionately related to tobacco use and exposure to tobacco smoke (Engeland *et al.* 1996). For other drugs with possible genotoxicity, such as dantron (a laxative), some anti-cancer drugs and some anti-retrovirals, while administration may be associated with an increased risk of cancer, there may be insufficient evidence to describe the adverse effect as dose-dependent in humans. For example, DNA changes in rodents and infants whose mothers received the anti-retroviral drugs zidovudine and lamivudine in pregnancy have not been associated with human cancers, to date (Poirier *et al.* 2004).

3

ADRs unrelated to dose (see chapter 21): Some of the rarest and most serious adverse events are unpredictable, idiosyncratic and may occur at any dose in any situation. They are not related to the known physiological actions of the drug, and include allergies or hypersentivity responses, such as drug rashes and anaphylaxis. They also include damage to major organs, such as liver or bone marrow. For example: liver and/or pancreatic failure arises in 1 in 37,000 adults taking valproate as monotherapy, and in 1 in 12,000 using the drug as part of a multidrug regimen; carbimazole causes a severe fall in white cell count (an allergic agranulocytosis) in 3 in 10,000 patients (Aronson 2006). While these adverse drug reactions are rare, they may guide patient monitoring.

Genetic variations influence vulnerability to idiosyncratic ADRs. Hearing loss following administration of gentamicin and related antibiotics may depend on genetic makeup. Some individuals are genetically vulnerable to drug-induced cardiac dysrhythmias associated with antipsychotics. People who inherit certain genetic conditions, such as porphyria (glossary) and glucose-6-phosphate dehydrogenase deficiency, are normally well, but may suddenly become very ill if they are administered certain drugs. Before administering the first dose of certain medications, e.g. oestrogens, mifepristone, sulphonamides, carbamazepine, ranitidine, it is prudent to ask for a family history of genetic conditions, as these drugs can trigger an acute attack of porphyria in susceptible people who may be unaware that they have inherited the condition (see BNF, section 9.8.2 for full list).

Withdrawal reactions:
Some drugs, such as corticosteroids, benzodiazepines, anti-depressants and beta blockers, may cause problems if they are abruptly discontinued after long-term use, and these 'withdrawal effects' may be described as adverse drug reactions (Edwards & Aronson 2000). Patients need support and monitoring during this time. If long-term medicines are to be discontinued, gradual withdrawal is usually advised, over several weeks, with patient monitoring. This can be expensive, in terms of practitioners' time.

Therapeutic failure:
Not all treatments are effective. For example only 2 in every 5 patients with moderate to severe pain have their pain reduced by 50% or more within 4–6 hours of administration of ibuprofen 400mg and 2 in 7 by 500mg paracetamol (Bandolier Extra 2003). Hypertension frequently does not respond to a single anti-hypertensive drug: a single anti-hypertensive agent typically lowers blood pressure by 7–8%, and a second drug is frequently needed (Williams *et al.* 2004). Sometimes, the underlying condition may worsen, and a therapy will cease to be effective, for example in asthma, diabetes or mental illness. Therefore, in many circumstances, patients benefit from ongoing monitoring of their original condition. More predictably, therapeutic failure may be induced by drug interactions. One important example is the prescription of carbamazepine or rifampicin to patients taking oral contraceptives.

Transgenerational adverse effects:
Transgenerational or second generation adverse drug reactions affect pregnancy, the fetus or the breastfed infant: the most notorious of these is thalidomide, but some familiar drugs, such as warfarin, anti-epileptic agents and lithium can also affect the fetus (BNF 2007). For many drugs and herbal remedies, manufacturers advise against use in pregnancy or during breastfeeding, on the grounds that there are insufficient human data to demonstrate safety. No drugs have been subjected to randomised controlled clinical trials to detect adverse effects in human pregnancy and lactation. Therefore, no drug has been demonstrated as 'safe'.

Drugs in pregnancy:
Drug-induced teratogenesis (glossary) is a result of cell damage. This is relevant to a wide variety of drugs, from alcohol to anti-cancer agents. If at all possible, drugs impairing cell division (such as anti-cancer drugs) should be avoided during the first 14–17 days of pregnancy, when they are most likely to cause abortion. The cells of the developing fetus are most vulnerable during the first trimester; however, the inner ear remains vulnerable beyond this time. Drugs impairing organ differentiation should be avoided between the 18th and 55th days of pregnancy, for example, lithium, oral anticoagulants. However, other drugs influence fetal development at later stages of pregnancy, for example, insulin, furosemide (frusemide), antithyroid agents. (See Jordan 2002b chapter 1 and appendix 4 of the BNF for fuller lists.)

The risk of fetal damage depends on several factors, as well as the chemical composition of the drug:

◆ stage of pregnancy
◆ amount of drug ingested
◆ number of doses: a single dose may be less damaging than repeated exposure
◆ Other agents to which mother and fetus are exposed

4

- mother's nutritional status
- genetic makeup of mother and fetus.

It is estimated that 4.8% of births and 4.0% of live births in Wales 1998–2003 were associated with a congenital anomaly (CARIS 2006). The causes of most, about two-thirds, congenital anomalies remain unknown, and less than 1% of congenital anomalies are attributable to prescribed drugs (Ruggiero 2006). Exposure of either parent to a medicinal product at any time during conception or pregnancy should be reported in association with congenital anomalies (ICH 1996). Currently, all reported congenital anomalies in Europe are reviewed by the PERISTAT project. In conjunction with EUROSTAT, this monitors perinatal health across Europe, and is able to detect abnormal clusters of problems (Macfarlane *et al.* 2003). However, attributing causation relies on data on prescribed medicines being accurately reported to those maintaining the databases. It is estimated that had data been collected more rigorously, the thalidomide tragedy would have been limited to 1,000 cases (Irl & Hasford 2000). The picture is complicated by epidemiological work which indicates that some congenital malformations, particularly cleft lip, cleft palate and congenital heart malformations, are associated with severe maternal stress during the first trimester of pregnancy (Hansen *et al.* 2000).

For some drugs, evidence of potential harm is gradually being accumulated from case series and retrospective analysis (see for example, McElhatton *et al.* 1999, Yoshida *et al.* 1999, Lattimore *et al.* 2005). Retrospective reporting of drug-induced fetal damage may lead to a bias towards over-reporting (Barzo *et al.* 1999), but this is often the only available data. However, years of experience with some drugs, such as paracetamol and penicillins, indicate that use at usual dosage is not manifestly harmful to the fetus. Women receiving long-term treatments should be helped to seek advice before conception or as soon as they realise they are pregnant. Some fetal abnormalities, including cardiac anomalies and neural tube defects, can be detected by screening early in pregnancy. It is sometimes possible for surgeons to correct defects before delivery: for example, heart valve defects caused by maternal lithium may be repaired *in utero*.

5

Drugs in childbirth:
Recently, it has been suggested that drugs given during childbirth could have long-term effects on the woman and baby. Antibiotics given during childbirth may alter the micro-organisms in the neonate's colon, which, in turn, might affect the regulation of the immune system, allowing development of allergy (Russell & Murch 2006). Also, opioid analgesics given in labour may pass into the baby, reducing its ability to coordinate and suckle correctly, painlessly and effectively; this reduces the chances of successful breastfeeding (Jordan *et al.* 2005, Jordan 2006). Women who have received high doses of analgesics in labour may need extra support over the first 1–3 days to establish breastfeeding. They may also be helped by informed explanations as to why they may be experiencing difficulties.

Breastfed infants:
Most drugs pass into breast milk, but the concentrations are sometimes too small to be harmful. For a few drugs, such as lithium or clozapine, there are reports of serious adverse reactions in infants. (Jordan 2002b chapter 1 and appendix 5 of the BNF have fuller lists.) For some medicines, there is relatively little information, and women who wish to breastfeed may need help to consult pharmacy information services.

1 Laxatives

A laxative is an agent that facilitates evacuation of the bowel.

Actions:

◆ Bulk laxatives such as bran, methylcellulose and ispaghula husk, stretch and stimulate the gastrointestinal tract.

◆ Osmotic laxatives (such as lactulose, magnesium sulphate (Epsom salts), macrogols, magnesium hydroxide mixture, phosphate enemas and sodium citrate enema) draw water into the gastrointestinal tract, thereby increasing the bulk of residue in the colon.

◆ Faecal softeners, such as liquid paraffin (not recommended), docusate sodium, mineral oils and arachis oil enema.

◆ Stimulant laxatives or purgatives are generally reserved for 'rescue therapy'. They irritate the gastrointestinal tract and include: senna, figs, rhubarb, castor oil (not recommended), bisacodyl, glycerol, dantron (carcinogenic in rodents, therefore use limited to terminal illness), docusate sodium and sodium picosulfate.

Indications:

◆ On initiation of **opioid** therapy when administration of opioids is expected to last more than five to seven days. Laxative therapy should not be delayed, as opioids predispose to gastrointestinal spasm and obstruction. In palliative care, stimulant laxatives are usually combined with faecal softeners or lactulose.

◆ If **straining** would exacerbate another condition, for example angina, anal fissure and haemorrhoids. Faecal softeners or bran or another bulk laxative are first choice (Courtenay & Butler 2000).

◆ Bowel investigations.

◆ Gastrointestinal disease, for example irritable bowel syndrome, diverticular disease and colostomy (bran or another bulk laxative is first choice).

◆ **Colonic constipation***, when:
   1. Serious pathology has been excluded, including gastrointestinal obstruction, cancers of the gastrointestinal tract, hypothyroidism, potassium deficiency.
   2. Drugs causing constipation have been reviewed or eliminated, as far as possible, for example, iron tablets, sedatives, non-prescription 'cold cures', opioids (including codeine in non-prescription cough medicines and analgesics), salbutamol, beta blockers, calcium channel blockers, some NSAIDs (not aspirin), some anti-emetics, most antipsychotics, some anti-depressants, aluminium-containing antacids, amphetamines (including ecstasy), cocaine, long-term laxatives, drugs causing dehydration, including diuretics and alcohol.
   3. Physiological measures have failed, for example: drinking one or two glasses of water with each meal, encouraging exercise, ensuring privacy, encouraging toileting immediately after meals, particularly breakfast, including more than 20g of dietary fibre/day in the diet. For example, each fruit and vegetable portion contains 2–4g of

dietary fibre. Beans and other legumes contain up to 8g fibre/serving. Bran cereal gives about 10g fibre/helping. Recommend five portions (15 ounces/375g) of fruit or vegetables daily.

◆ Management of faecal incontinence, due to dementia, decreased storage capacity or overflow, may involve controlled defecation twice weekly (Wald 2007).

◆ Failure to pass faeces within three days of childbirth (single dose).

◆ Lactulose is prescribed in advanced **liver disease** to minimise the associated central nervous system disturbances (known as hepatic encephalopathy). Doses are usually higher than those prescribed for constipation.

* Colonic constipation may be defined as a delay in the passage of food residue due to the accumulation of hard, dry stool, associated with painful defecation, abdominal distension and a palpable mass. The frequency of bowel evacuation varies with the individual: once every three days is a minimum.

Administration: Administer with a full glass of water or other liquid, particularly bulk laxatives (Food and Drug Administration 2007). See Box 1.1. For patients who have not previously taken laxatives, use the lowest possible dose.

Box 1.1 Oral administration of medications

◆ Practitioners avoid touching medicines, if possible (Railton 2007).

◆ Gloves are worn when handling drugs which could be absorbed through the skin (e.g. creams, transdermal patches, anti-cancer drugs, nitrates) or cause irritation and contact dermatitis (e.g. chlorpromazine) (Smith *et al.* 2008).

◆ Medicines should be swallowed with a full glass of water.

◆ The patient should sit upright, and remain upright for 30 minutes (McKenry & Salerno 2003).

◆ Liquid formulations are usually absorbed more rapidly than solids.

◆ Older adults may find liquids difficult to swallow, and prefer to take orodispersible preparations with soft food, such as puddings.

◆ **Crushing tablets** usually hastens absorption and damages any coatings; this may cause adverse effects. If a tablet is crushed or a capsule is opened, fine particles may be released into the air (see antibacterials, cytotoxics).

◆ The effect of food on drug absorption should be checked (Schmidt & Dalhoff 2002, Jordan *et al.* 2003). A consistent relation to meals is usually advised. Food may:
  ❖ prevent drug-induced nausea,
  ❖ reduce the rate of drug absorption (see table 15.2).

◆ Modified release tablets should not be broken, crushed or chewed.

For administration *via* enteral feeding tubes see BAPEN (2003), Jordan *et al.* (2003), Chan (2002), Thomson *et al.* (2000), Naysmith and Nicholson (1998).

Separate administration from other drugs and food by 1–2 hours, if possible. If the patient finds the sweet taste of lactulose unduly unpleasant, administration with fruit juice may make it more palatable. Magnesium hydroxide mixture is stored outside a refrigerator.

Bulk laxatives should not be administered before retiring. They should also never be administered into enteral feeding tubes because they expand on contact with moisture and block the tubes.

If the patient has faecal impaction, avoid oral laxatives, as overflow diarrhoea, with faecal incontinence, may occur. Suppositories or enemas may be prescribed.

Rectal administration is best avoided for patients with haemorrhoids or anal fissure. Glycerol suppositories should not be handled because they dissolve at body temperature. See Box 1.2.

Box 1.2 Rectal administration of medications

Check:

◆ Risk of infection, particularly patients with impaired immunity.

◆ Risk of bleeding, particularly patients prescribed anticoagulants.

◆ Signs of irritation, particularly with repeated use of carbamazepine, NSAIDs.

◆ Insertion is above the anal sphincter. This can be identified by asking the client to 'bear down'. The suppository should be inserted some 1.5 inches above this.

◆ Patient remains lying for 15 minutes. Reassess after 15 minutes.

◆ Signs and symptoms of both over- and under-dosing. Absorption is unpredictable, due to:
  ❖ Presence/ absence of faeces.
  ❖ Uncertain positioning of suppository.

Avoid rectal administration if patient has:

◆ recent prostate, rectal or colon surgery.

◆ high risk of infection or bleeding.

◆ cardiac dysrhythmias (irregularities) or recent heart attack. Heart rate may fall.

◆ undiagnosed abdominal pain. Increased peristalsis could worsen any obstruction or rupture an inflamed appendix.

(Hayes *et al*. 2003, Wilkinson 2001, Holmer Pettersson *et al*. 2006, Smith *et al*. 2008)

The delay between laxative administration and bowel movement varies with preparation (Table 1.1). Laxatives acting in 6–12 hours are best taken before going to bed. If the first dose is given in the daytime, the patient may experience faecal incontinence at night. However, short-acting magnesium compounds are best administered in the morning.

Table 1.1 Usual timing of laxative action

1–3 Days	6–12 Hours	1–4 Hours
Bulking agents	Senna	Magnesium sulphate
Lactulose	Bisacodyl	Phosphate or sodium enemas
Docusate sodium	Sodium picosulfate	Castor oil
	Codanthramer	Bisacodyl suppository

Note: These timings relate to adults. Some laxatives, for example senna, act more rapidly in children

Drugs which take one to three days to work should be used for prevention and not on an 'as required' or 'rescue' basis.

Adverse effects: implications for practice

Stimulation of defecation may cause diarrhoea. Excessive loss of water and electrolytes may ensue. In dehydrated, debilitated patients, bulk laxatives may swell on ingestion and obstruct the gastrointestinal tract.

Potential Problem	Suggestions for Prevention and Management
Flatulence and diarrhoea or nausea	Stop laxative/reduce dose. Consider the possibility that lactulose has been administered to a patient with 'lactose intolerance' (glossary).
Loss of appetite/feeling full	Monitor food intake in older people (mainly bulk laxatives).
Abdominal cramps/colic, due to excessive gastrointestinal contractions	Consider the possibility of gastrointestinal obstruction. Discuss, with prescriber, reducing dose or discontinuing.
Dehydration (particularly osmotic laxatives). This may be due to diarrhoea. Gastrointestinal obstruction	Take with full glass of water. Monitor fluid balance if patient is debilitated. On a normal diet about 5 glasses/cups of liquid should be drunk (see diuretics).
Choking	Avoid bulk laxatives before retiring.
Electrolyte disturbance, associated with laxative abuse	Limit use to one to two weeks. If this is not possible, monitor potassium concentration in venous blood samples. Particularly if: ◆ Other drugs lowering potassium and magnesium are administered – for example, diuretics. ◆ Other drugs increase the risks of cardiac arrhythmias/dysrhythmias – for example, antipsychotics and antidepressants. ◆ There is a history of laxative abuse or eating disorders. It is not appropriate to monitor venous blood samples in some circumstances, such as palliative care. Ask patients to report cramps, weakness or dizziness (symptoms of hypokalaemia). Encourage foods rich in potassium, such as raisins, meat, bananas and oranges.
Loss of minerals and protein	Bulk laxatives may reduce absorption of iron, calcium and zinc. If use is prolonged, monitor full blood count. Encourage a balanced diet.
Fluid retention due to sodium content	Avoid laxatives with high sodium content. For example, each 13.8gram sachet of Movicol® contains macrogol, and some 200mg sodium, and up to 8 can be taken in a day to treat faecal impaction (ABPI 2007). (Recommended maximum daily sodium intake is 2.4grams (RCP/BHS 2006).) Particular care for patients with heart failure or hypertension.

Absorption of magnesium	Avoid magnesium salts in debilitated patients, and those with liver or kidney failure. This can cause cardiac dysrhythmias.
Laxative dependence and atonic colon	If possible, restrict use to one to two weeks. Continued use may damage the colonic reflexes. Advise patients that, following complete evacuation, further bowel movements may not occur for up to two days.
Urine discolouration	Warn patients that this harmless reaction may occur with senna and other stimulant laxatives.
Rectal irritation	Discontinue, if advised by prescriber. (Bisacodyl suppositories)
Aggravation of haemorrhoids or anal fissures	Review laxative use. Avoid rectal administration, particularly docusate preparations.
Throat irritation	Avoid liquid formulations, such as liquid docusate.
Therapeutic failure	Monitor output and girth, to detect obstruction as early as possible. Check fluid balance. Be prepared to administer suppositories or enemas, as advised. Review diet to ensure that foods promoting constipation are minimised e.g. hard boiled eggs, rice, high-sugar foods, processed cheese.

Cautions and contra-indications:

- Avoid prolonged use, particularly stimulant laxatives, if possible.
- **Pregnancy**: stimulant laxatives are best avoided. Castor oil has been known to stimulate uterine contractions. Manufacturers of Dulcolax® advise to avoid during pregnancy. Manufacturers of Senokot® advise use of syrup preparations only. Bulk laxatives are regarded as safe. Use of laxatives is best restricted to single doses (Courtenay and Butler 2000).
- **Breastfeeding**: senna is excreted into breastmilk (Pasricha 2006), but is not known to be harmful (BNF 2007).
- **Children**: seek medical advice. Manufacturers do no recommend senna for children under 6.
- **Older adults**: reduce initial dose. For example, 7.5mg senna may be more than sufficient in the laxative-naïve patient.

Laxatives are not advised for patients with certain conditions:

- Obstruction of the gastrointestinal tract (a particular risk if opioids have been initiated).
- Atonic, flacid colon.
- Eating disorders (predispose to laxative abuse).
- Debility: dehydration will be worsened. Impaction in the oesophagus is possible if bran or figs are given without adequate water to older, dehydrated patients.

◆ Avoid dantron if faecal incontinence is possible, as prolonged contact of dantron with the skin causes irritation or excoriation.

Check product information for patients with:

◆ **Diabetes** – some bulk laxatives, such as Normacol®, contain carbohydrate, such as sucrose or maltodextrin, and lactulose contains galactose, which may raise blood sugar (Aronson 2006, McKenry & Salerno 2003). Ensure blood glucose concentrations are monitored regularly.

◆ Galactosaemia - lactulose worsens this rare condition.

◆ Phenylketonuria – some preparations, such as Fybogel® and Ispagel Orange®, contain aspartame, which worsens this rare condition.

◆ Patients with **colostomies or ileostomies** may lose considerable volumes of fluid if administered osmotic laxatives, such as magnesium citrate.

◆ Patients with **swallowing difficulties** are at increased risk of choking or oesophageal obstruction if prescribed bulk laxatives (Food and Drug Administration 2007).

Interactions (summary):

◆ Loss of other drugs due to diarrhoea.

◆ Bulk laxatives impair absorption of some drugs and minerals.

◆ Increased risk of potassium depletion with co-administration of: beta$_2$ agonists, diuretics, digoxin, corticosteroids, liquorice.

◆ Increased risk of dehydration.

◆ Co-administration of enteric coated stimulant laxatives with antacids or proton-pump inhibitors may cause stomach cramps.

2 Controlling Gastric Acidity

Excess gastric acidity not only causes pain and discomfort, but can lead to gastric erosion and, in acute settings, lung damage. Several different drugs reduce these problems.

Actions: Excess gastric acidity may be relieved by:

◆ **Antacids**, such as aluminium hydroxide, magnesium carbonate, are alkaline compounds that react with acids to form neutral compounds.

◆ **Barrier compounds**, for example alginates, sucralfate, form a physical layer between the acid in the stomach and the lining of the gastrointestinal (GI) tract. Compound preparations e.g. Gaviscon Advance®, Rennie Duo® contain both antacids and barrier compounds.

◆ **Prostaglandin** analogues, such as misoprostol, strengthen the protective lining of the GI tract.

◆ **Histamine$_2$-receptor antagonists** (H$_2$RAs), for example ranitidine, famotidine, modify acid production by blocking the stimulatory effects of histamine.

◆ **Proton-pump inhibitors** (PPIs), for example omeprazole, lansoprazole, pantoprazole, inhibit acid formation in the cells lining the stomach. These are the most powerful acid suppressants.

Indications: Reducing acidity alleviates pain and/or prevents tissue damage in:

◆ **Indigestion**, when lifestyle modifications have failed. These include: sleeping on left side; avoiding food for two hours before lying down; avoiding irritants (cola, coffee, tea, alcohol, smoking, citrus & tomato juices) and high-fat foods (including chocolate); smaller meals; raising the height of the bed-head. Prescription of drugs known to irritate the oesophagus should be reviewed, for example: clindamycin, doxycycline, tetracycline, iron, NSAIDs and bisphosphonates, such as alendronate.

◆ **Gastro-oesophageal reflux disease** (GORD/GERD), when medications which exacerbate the condition have been reviewed, particularly: sedatives; calcium channel blockers; nitrates; anti-muscarinics; some antipsychotics; theophylline; tricyclic antidepressants (Katz 2003).

◆ **Gastric and duodenal ulceration**. Tests for *Helicobacter pylori* should be undertaken, as eradication regimens are often effective. If *Helicobacter pylori* is not eradicated, ulcers are likely to recur. Any use of non-steroidal anti-inflammatory drugs (NSAIDs) should be reviewed. In acute settings, H$_2$RAs are administered to prevent 'stress induced ulcers'. These are attributed to prolonged activation of the sympathetic nervous system, which diverts blood from the rest of the body to heart, brain and lungs, disrupting the blood supply to the gut wall and leaving the lining vulnerable.

◆ **NSAID-induced ulcers** or prophylaxis when NSAIDs cannot be withdrawn.

◆ Anaesthesia and sedation. The risk of lung damage associated with aspiration of gastric contents is reduced.

◆ Zollinger-Elinson syndrome (over-production of the hormone gastrin).

◆ Anti-cancer treatments and cystic fibrosis. PPIs may prevent or control symptoms.

◆ Alcohol-induced gastritis (unlicensed).

Administration: Where possible, administration is restricted to 4- to 8-week courses.

◆ **Antacids** are intended for short-term symptom relief. Magnesium and sodium compounds give almost immediate relief, but aluminium takes longer. Antacids work for about 30 minutes if taken on an empty stomach, but remain effective for several hours when administered after food. Usual doses are 5–10ml of liquid or one to two tablets up to four times per day. Chewable tablets must be thoroughly masticated and followed by a glass of water. Suspensions work more quickly than tablets (Hoogerwerf & Pasricha 2006).

◆ **H$_2$RAs** are most effective when taken on an empty stomach, at bedtime. H$_2$RAs are also administered intravenously.

◆ **PPIs** are usually administered once daily, 30 minutes before breakfast; the contents of some capsules can be mixed with water, fruit juice or yoghurt. Lansoprazole tablets can be placed on the tongue for rapid absorption and symptom relief. Some PPIs can be administered intravenously. The effects of PPIs last for 48 hours after the last dose.

◆ **Misoprostol** is administered with meals and NSAIDs.

Adverse effects: In excess, gastric acid damages the lining of the GI tract. However, it is important for killing ingested micro-organisms, digesting protein and absorbing iron and vitamin B$_{12}$.

ALL ACID SUPPRESSANTS MAY CAUSE:

◆ **Gastrointestinal problems.** Altered bowel movements are common, and largely predictable.

◆ **Loss of acidity (**unlikely with antacids**)**
  ❖ Without gastric acid, the number of micro-organisms in the upper GI tract increases, and **infections** are more likely. There is no absolute barrier separating the GI tract from the lungs. Fluid from the stomach enters the respiratory tract, *via* the pharynx. Normally, the cilia lining the respiratory tract prevent significant quantities of GI tract secretions reaching the air sacs and alveoli. If the gastrointestinal secretions are not first sterilised by stomach acid, they are more likely to infect the lungs.
  ❖ Absorption of vitamin B$_{12}$ and iron requires gastric acid. If therapy continues for several months, B$_{12}$ stores may become low and anaemia or nerve damage may result.

Misoprostol is a prostaglandin. It causes contraction of the smooth muscle of the GI tract and uterus, and dilates the blood vessels.

13

Adverse effects: implications for practice: ACID SUPPRESSANTS

Potential Problem	Suggestions for Prevention and Management
Gastrointestinal problems	
Constipation (sucralfate, aluminium compounds and PPIs)	Changing medication may be effective. Encourage mobility, fluid intake, high fibre/fruit diet and monitoring of bowel movements.
Diarrhoea/flatulence (magnesium compounds, misoprostol and H$_2$RAs)	Prompt rehydration. Monitor electrolytes for potassium loss if diarrhoea is severe or persistent. Restrict misoprostol to 200mg/day. Many patients discontinue misoprostol because of diarrhoea and colic. If this has been prescribed to protect against NSAID-induced ulcers, monitor compliance, and seek more convenient therapy, if necessary. Stool culture to exclude infection, if indicated.
Dry or sore mouth	Patients receiving intensive care require meticulous mouth care. Offer ice cubes or sips of water.
Abdominal pain, distension and vomiting (misoprostol and PPIs)	Exclude serious cause, including liver or pancreatic damage. Reduce dose or change acid suppressant.
Bezoar (a fibrous mass formed in the stomach from ingested food or hair) formation and gastrointestinal obstruction	Avoid administration of sucralfate or alginates within one hour of enteral feeds. Cautious use of sucralfate in seriously ill patients or if gastric emptying is delayed.
Loss of acidity	
Gastrointestinal infections: **Salmonella** **Possible association with *Clostridium difficile* in hospitalised patients receiving antibiotic therapy**	Advice regarding food hygiene. Early recognition is important to prevent dehydration and electrolyte imbalance.
Respiratory infections Particularly in ventilated patients (sucralfate is relatively free of this problem)	In high risk areas, monitor temperature and lung bases. Adopt semi-recumbent position, if possible. Advise primary care patients regarding symptoms and seeking advice.

14

Anaemia or Vitamin B$_{12}$ deficiency	Monitor full blood count and B$_{12}$ concentrations yearly with long-term use.
Vitamin B$_{12}$ concentrations decline in 33% (15/49) patients on long-term PPI therapy (Schenk et al. 1999); less risk with H$_2$RAs	Administer oral B$_{12}$ supplements, if necessary. Vegetarians should be monitored for iron-deficiency.
Therapeutic failure	
Worsening symptoms **Calcium ions in a number of preparations (e.g. Gaviscon Advance®) stimulate gastric acid release, which intensifies, rather than alleviates, symptoms** **Sodium bicarbonate reacts with gastric acid to produce carbon dioxide and the subsequent gastric distension increases acid production**	Avoid preparations containing calcium or sodium bicarbonate. If symptoms persist, foods containing calcium should be avoided, and alternative therapy sought.
Increased reflux symptoms	Be aware this may occur following eradication of *Helicobacter pylori* or abrupt withdrawal of PPIs.
Persistent symptoms	Advise patients that PPIs may take 2–5 days to achieve full benefit. Take PPI before both breakfast and evening meal to avoid nocturnal symptoms (Katz 2003).

 ## Additional adverse effects: implications for practice: misoprostol, PPIs, H$_2$RAs

Potential Problem	Suggestions for Prevention and Management
Cardiovascular system	
Hypotension/postural hypotension (misoprostol only)	Check BP lying and standing for older patients (see diuretics).
Bradycardia, cardiac dysrhythmias and postural hypotension when administering H$_2$RAs intravenously	Dilute dose and administer over at least 10 minutes. Gradual infusions over longer periods are recommended.

Neurological effects	
Headache, tiredness, dizziness, paraesthesia, rarely confusion, hallucinations, depression and involuntary movements (very rare) H₂RAs block the neurotransmitter histamine, which affects nerve function	Recognise and report problems, particularly in seriously ill, older patients. Problems reverse on discontinuation.
Visual impairment (PPI injections only)	Administer injections slowly.
Endocrine disruption	
Impotence Cimetidine (occasionally ranitidine or lansoprazole) in high doses blocks the actions of testosterone leading to breast development	Discuss with same-gender nurse. Alternative therapy may be advised.

16 Rare adverse effects include: rashes, fever, muscle or joint pain, hair loss, damage to liver or pancreas, nephritis, anaphylaxis, blood disorders. Raised triglycerides with long-term pantoprazole.

ADDITIONAL ADVERSE EFFECTS: IMPLICATIONS FOR PRACTICE: ANTACIDS

ABSORPTION OF MINERALS

◆ **Calcium.** Some 15% of oral calcium is absorbed. Excess calcium and magnesium appears in urine, where it can form kidney stones or deposits on urinary catheters. In patients without catheters, this is problematic if large quantities of antacids and calcium compounds (2–3g of calcium carbonate) or dairy products are taken (Kaklamanos and Perros 2007). However, lower doses contain sufficient minerals and alkali to block urinary catheters (Burr & Nuseibeh 1997).

◆ **Sodium.** Regular use of antacids may result in more sodium being ingested than can be eliminated. Sodium retention leads to fluid retention, which can cause or exacerbate heart failure and hypertension.

◆ **Aluminium long-term** reduces absorption of phosphates, which affects bone density.

Potential Problem	Suggestions for Prevention and Management
Absorption of sodium	
Breathlessness and oedema, (sodium-containing preparations)	Monitor older patients for weakness and fluid retention (see beta blockers). Substitute sodium-free products for patients with hypertension, heart, liver or renal problems, however mild.
Absorption of calcium	
Blocked catheters, particularly patients with low fluid intake	Patients with indwelling urinary catheters should avoid antacids, effervescent tablets and excess intake of citrate to minimise risk of blockage.
Renal colic and/or hypercalcaemia (rare)	Review antacid therapy.
Long-term ingestion of aluminium	
Bone weakness	Monitor serum phosphate concentrations with regular aluminium administration, particularly for patients with renal impairment.

Cautions and contra-indications:

◆ **Renal Impairment.** Antacids, particularly effervescent formulations, should be restricted because magnesium, potassium, sodium and aluminium may accumulate and affect the heart. Doses of pantoprazole and most H_2RAs should be reduced.

◆ **Heart failure and hypertension** can be caused or worsened by preparations containing sodium, which should be avoided by all patients on sodium-restricted diets. Gaviscon® Advance tablets contain 47mg sodium, and Peptac® suspension contains 71mg sodium/5ml. (BNF 2007) The maximum 80ml/day of Peptac® suspension gives a sodium intake almost half the recommended daily allowance (2.4g).

◆ **Cardiovascular and cerebrovascular disease** may be worsened by misoprostol-induced postural hypotension.

◆ **Diabetes.** Some preparations may contain significant quantities of glucose.

◆ **Hepatic impairment.** Avoid antacids containing sodium or causing constipation. Low doses of PPIs or H_2RAs may be prescribed.

◆ **Tube feeding.** Antacids are best avoided. They may interact with enteral feeds, thereby blocking the tubes.

◆ **Inflammatory bowel disease** may be worsened by misoprostol.

◆ **2 weeks before tests for** *Helicobacter pylori:* avoid PPIs and H_2RAs.

◆ **Pregnancy.**

  ❖ Misoprostol is contra-indicated in pregnancy and women planning pregnancy. It stimulates uterine contractions and induces abortion. (This is an unlicensed use.)

❖ PPIs reported as fetotoxic in animal studies. Manufacturers advise to avoid.

❖ H$_2$RAs are used safely during childbirth. Manufacturers advise to avoid if possible during pregnancy.

❖ Antacids, used occasionally, are regarded as safe. Minimise doses of sodium and calcium.

◆ **Breastfeeding.** Little information is available, therefore manufacturers advise to avoid. Occasional use of antacids regarded as safe.

◆ **Porphyria** (glossary). Ranitidine should be avoided.

It has been suggested that long-term suppression of gastric acidity could increase the risk of gastric cancer. While there is no evidence that this has happened, a few patients taking long-term PPIs have developed gastric polyps. Therefore, *Helicobacter pylori* is eradicated before long-term therapy is started (Aronson 2006).

Interactions (summary): Many acid suppressants can be bought without prescription. When taking 'drug histories', nurses should specifically inquire about these products as they interact with many medications.

Acid suppressants reduce absorption of iron, some ampicillin preparations, ketoconazole and itraconazole.

Antacids should be administered two hours apart from other drugs as they may impair or enhance absorption and damage enteric coatings. This causes premature release of the enteric-coated drug. If preparations containing levodopa are co-administered, the control of Parkinson's disease should be monitored. Antacids increase excretion of aspirin and aminoglycoside antibiotics, thereby jeopardising clinical efficacy (Wallace & Amsden 2002). Antacids containing sodium (most antacids) can significantly reduce lithium concentrations, precipitating a relapse of mental illness and, therefore, should be avoided in patients prescribed lithium.

PPIs may impair elimination of several drugs. This is most relevant with warfarin and phenytoin.

Cimetidine inhibits the elimination of many drugs, including amitriptyline, amiodarone, valproate, phenytoin, warfarin and ciclosporin; these interactions are important, and co-administration is best avoided. Other H$_2$RAs interact with fewer drugs.

Contributor

David Gallimore BSc, MSc, RGN. Tutor in Adult Nursing at the School of Health Sciences, University of Wales, Swansea

3 Diuretics

Diuretics increase the volume of urine passed and decrease the volume of fluid in the circulation (Rang *et al.* 2007).

Commonly prescribed diuretics include:
◆ loop diuretics (furosemide/frusemide, bumetanide)
◆ thiazides (bendroflumethiazide/bendrofluazide, chlortalidone, indapamide)
◆ potassium-sparing diuretics (amiloride, triamterene), including aldosterone antagonists (spironolactone, eplerenone).

Actions: Together, these are known as the 'transport-inhibiting diuretics' because they block the enzymes which reabsorb electrolytes (sodium, potassium and chloride) from urine into the circulation. As electrolytes are lost in the urine, water is lost with them. This does not work so well if the patient takes a high salt diet or smokes. Diuretics also dilate blood vessels.

Each group of diuretics has its own site of action (Figure 3.1):

◆ Loop diuretics are the most powerful because they block enzymes in the Loop of Henle, which is responsible for reabsorption of up to 25% water and electrolytes from urine back into the circulation.

◆ Thiazides act in the distal convoluted tubules, which reabsorb up to 10% water and electrolytes. Therefore, thaizides usually induce a smaller diuresis.

◆ Potassium-sparing diuretics act on the collecting tubules and block potassium loss.

Indications: Diuretics are prescribed when the body contains too much fluid. This occurs in hypertension and conditions associated with oedema, such as cirrhosis, nephrotic syndrome, chronic renal failure, and acute and chronic congestive heart failure. Thiazide diuretics may be the initial choice of therapy for hypertension (RCP/BHS 2006, NICE 2006a). For 'swollen ankles', physiological measures, such as exercise and resting with legs elevated, are the preferred treatment (BNF 2007).

◆ **Loop diuretics:** acute therapy: pulmonary oedema, renal failure; long term: heart failure, occasionally hypertension.

◆ **Thiazides and related drugs:** long term: hypertension, heart failure, oedema.

◆ **Potassium-sparing diuretics** are prescribed with other diuretics to reduce potassium loss.

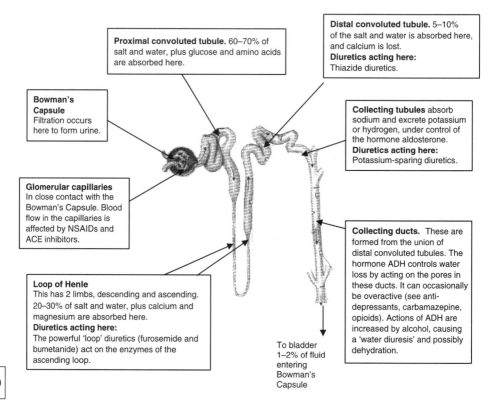

Proximal convoluted tubule. 60–70% of salt and water, plus glucose and amino acids are absorbed here.

Distal convoluted tubule. 5–10% of the salt and water is absorbed here, and calcium is lost.
Diuretics acting here: Thiazide diuretics.

Bowman's Capsule Filtration occurs here to form urine.

Collecting tubules absorb sodium and excrete potassium or hydrogen, under control of the hormone aldosterone.
Diuretics acting here: Potassium-sparing diuretics.

Glomerular capillaries In close contact with the Bowman's Capsule. Blood flow in the capillaries is affected by NSAIDs and ACE inhibitors.

Collecting ducts. These are formed from the union of distal convoluted tubules. The hormone ADH controls water loss by acting on the pores in these ducts. It can occasionally be overactive (see anti-depressants, carbamazepine, opioids). Actions of ADH are increased by alcohol, causing a 'water diuresis' and possibly dehydration.

Loop of Henle This has 2 limbs, descending and ascending. 20–30% of salt and water, plus calcium and magnesium are absorbed here.
Diuretics acting here: The powerful 'loop' diuretics (furosemide and bumetanide) act on the enzymes of the ascending loop.

To bladder 1–2% of fluid entering Bowman's Capsule

Each kidney contains one million nephrons or renal units. The kidneys control salt and water balance and eliminate waste products to maintain a stable internal environment for the rest of the body. The functioning of the kidneys can be considered as two processes:
- glomerular filtration rate (GFR) (which takes place in the Bowman's Capsule)
- tubular secretion and reabsorption

Figure 3.1   Drugs acting on the nephron

Administration: Oral administration should be linked to meal-times, to reduce any gastrointestinal upsets. Food may reduce furosemide-induced diuresis (Baxter 2006), therefore a consistent relationship to meals may be advisable. Absorption of bumetanide or torasemide is less unpredictable (Jackson 2006a). If heart failure worsens, absorption may decrease, making the diuretic less effective.

Most thiazides induce a diuresis within 1–2 hours; this lasts 12–24 hours. Therefore, thiazides are usually administered in the morning.

Oral furosemide induces diuresis within 1 hour and diuresis continues for 6 hours. Administration <6 hours before bedtime may disturb sleep. Discuss with patient the most convenient time for administration and suggest flexibility to accommodate social engagements.

Intravenous furosemide acts within 20–60 minutes. Rapid administration (>4mg/minutes) risks damage to hearing and balance.

Elderly patients receive lower initial doses, which are subsequently adjusted according to kidney function tests (serum creatinine and glomerular filtration rate (GFR), chapter 21).

Adverse effects:

◆ **Loss of salt and water from tissues and circulation into urine.** Problems will be intensified by other causes of fluid depletion e.g. fever, gastrointestinal upset, reduction in intake of food or fluid.

◆ **Loss of potassium, magnesium and hydrogen ions** occurs as reabsorption from urine is blocked by loop diuretics. Thiazide and loop diuretics increase the amount of sodium entering the distal tubules. As the enzymes attempt to reabsorb this, they lose excessive amounts of potassium. Where there is a shortage of potassium ions, hydrogen ions may be lost instead. This upsets the acid/base balance. Potassium sparing diuretics counter this, but can cause potassium retention.

◆ Long-standing potassium deficiency may lead to reduced insulin secretion and hyperglycaemia (Zillich *et al.* 2006).

◆ **Hyperuricaemia** (accumulation of uric acid) may occur when the volumes of fluid entering the kidney tubules are low, causing gout.

◆ Calcium imbalance, impotence, damage to inner ear.

Adverse effects: implications for practice: Regular reviews of vital signs, blood biochemistry and medication are necessary, pre-therapy and at least annually (Aronson 2006). Problems are most likely to arise with higher doses.

Potential Problem	Suggestions for Prevention and Management
Loss of salt and water	
Excessive diuresis (>100ml/hour) may lead to functional incontinence	Establish dose schedule that minimises inconvenience.
	Ensure commode or bedpans nearby; provide privacy.
	Monitor residual urine volume to assess any urine retention, particularly in older men who may have prostatic enlargement. Continue to monitor urine volume once heart failure has been treated, as diuretic dose may become excessive when oedema has resolved.
	Advise patients of the impact of cold weather on continence control.
	If diuresis is affecting quality of life or causing retention of urine, and dose reduction is not possible, discuss the possibility of substituting chlortalidone (taken alternate days) for other thiazides. This may 'normalise' micturition patterns, due to its longer half-life (47 hours) (glossary).
With high doses, risk of circulatory collapse (particularly loop diuretics)	In **acute care,** assess urinary output, fluid balance and vital signs frequently for rapid changes.
	Administer intravenous injections slowly.
	Weigh clients before therapy and daily. Weigh under standard conditions: early morning before eating or drinking, after urination, with same amount of clothing and using same scales in the same place. Report changes greater than 1kg (2.2lb)/day.

Hypotension and orthostatic/postural hypotension	Record BP before therapy and 2–4 times daily in acute setting. Systolic BP<100mmHg indicates hypotension.
	Measure BP lying/sitting and standing; 1 minute should elapse between the 2 measurements: a fall in systolic BP >20mmHg (Bennett 1994) or 10% indicates orthostatic hypotension (Berg 1999).
	Instruct client to stand slowly. Assess carefully before assisting with mobility.
	Advise patients to avoid long periods of standing, hot showers and exposure to hot environments.
Dehydration	Ensure adequate fluid intake: 35ml/kg body weight for adults, plus any abnormal loss. About 1000–1300ml of this is normally taken in from foods, leaving about 1000–1500ml to be taken as about 5 glasses of cups of fluid (Howard 2001). Excessive water restriction may cause rebound fluid retention.
	Monitor heart rate lying/sitting and standing: a rise of 10% on standing indicates dehydration (Berg 1999).
	Check urea and creatinine concentrations.

Consequences of dehydration:	
Dry mouth, stomatitis	Frequent mouth rinses. Monitor oral cavity for caries and ulcers.
Constipation	Maintain fluid intake, high fibre diet and moderate exercise, if not contraindicated. Monitor bowel movements; if <2/week review intake of fruit and fibre.
Hearing impairment due to hardening and impaction of ear wax	Monitor hearing, particularly in older men, when diuretics are commenced. Arrange for examination of the external auditory meatus. Removal of wax reverses hearing loss.
Vision disturbance	If problems persist after first few weeks, seek advice.
Increased risk of thrombosis	Check haematocrit (glossary). If raised (>47% women, 54% men), report to prescriber. Increased fluid intake may be needed.
Hyponatraemia (glossary) **Sodium loss may occasionally be excessive, reducing sodium concentrations below normal** **Headache, lethargy, anorexia, nausea and vomiting may be early signs**	Monitor sodium concentrations, together with potassium, because serious deficits can arise without symptoms. Maximum risk: ◆ thiazides first 1–14 days of therapy ◆ loop diuretics within 6 months of initiation Report urgently and withhold if serum sodium<130 mmol/l. Values <120 mmol/l have been associated with neurological damage.

Loss of potassium, magnesium and hydrogen ions	
Hypokalaemia (glossary) (potassium concentration <3.5 mmol/l) may cause a range of problems from vague symptoms of weakness to sudden cardiac events (thiazides and loop diuretics)	Monitor serum potassium pre-therapy, regularly and if diarrhoea or vomiting occur. If <4.0 mmol/l report to prescriber and discuss potassium-sparing diuretics (Zillich *et al.* 2006). Particular care if patient has a colostomy/ileostomy. Monitor ECG. Be alert for palpitations, fatigue, depression, constipation or cramps. Cardiac problems are intensified if patient is hypoxic. Advise clients to eat potassium-rich foods, such as bananas, raisins, oranges, orange juice, meat (Karch 2006). Avoid potassium supplements if possible. Particular care in patients with heart failure and muscle wasting.
Hypomagnesaemia	A healthy diet containing wholegrain foods and green vegetables gives an adequate supply of magnesium.
Acid/base disturbances **At high doses, loss of hydrogen ions disrupts the body's acid/base balance and causes metabolic alkalosis**	In acute care, doctors review acid/base status regularly. In continuing care, changes in acidity or alkalinity of urine may predispose to urinary tract infection. Monitoring urine for possible infection will also aid in continence control and catheter care. Encourage clear fluids. Check bladder for residual urine.
Hyperglycaemia Diabetes in 11.6% of patients after 4 years (1–3% above incidence with other antihyperensives) (ALLHAT 2002) **Mainly thiazides**	Monitor blood glucose regularly, including 4 & 8 weeks after initiation or dose increase. Follow up must be indefinite. Seek medical advice, if >5.6 mmol/l, as this may indicate increased risk of diabetes (Genuth *et al.* 2003) or, if >6.0 mmol/l, cardiovascular event (Balkau *et al.* 1998). Ensure diuretic dose is kept to the minimum necessary. Be prepared to increase dose of any anti-diabetic agents.
Increased cholesterol and triglyceride concentrations	Monitor lipid profile pre-therapy & 3–6 months after initiation (Aronson 2006). If adversely affected, suggest reduction in dietary fat or seek alternative therapy for hypertension. Ensure diuretic dose is kept to minimum necessary.
Calcium imbalance	
Hypercalcaemia Thiazide diuretics increase absorption of calcium from urine **Risk of osteoporosis may be reduced**	Be prepared to monitor calcium concentrations. Discontinue thiazides before performing parathyroid function tests. Avoid calcium and vitamin D supplements.
Hypocalcaemia Loop diuretics block reabsorption of calcium ions	Increased risk of osteoporosis with long-term loop diuretics. Consider calcium and vitamin D supplements. Maintain high fluid intake to reduce risk of renal calculi. With high doses, be alert for tetany.

Hyperuricaemia	
Gout, Particular risk in men >90kg prescribed thiazides and intaking >56 units alcohol/week	Be aware that joint pain, particularly neck pain, may indicate diuretic-induced gout. Monitor uric acid concentrations.

Impotence	
Male impotence (prevalence between 3–32%) may be due to changes in blood vessels Spironolactone causes gynaecomastia and impotence	Discuss with same-gender nurse. If appropriate, record history pre-therapy. Discuss possible dose reduction or medication review with prescriber. If appropriate, advise patients of associations with age, hypertension, diabetes and antihypertensives.

Inner ear	
Impaired hearing and balance (loop diuretics) usually reversible. An enzyme similar to that in the Loop of Henle controls fluid balance in the inner ear	Monitor, particularly with intravenous administration. Mobilise carefully. Ask patient to report any tinnitus. Report to prescriber. If therapy is not discontinued, permanent deafness could follow.

Hyperkalaemia	
Potassium accumulation is a risk with potassium-sparing diuretics	Potassium must be monitored carefully in: older patients, patients receiving blood transfusion, with diabetes, AIDS or any degree of renal impairment (serum creatinine >130micromol/l). Advise against ingesting potassium supplements or salt substitutes, which usually contain potassium, or large amounts of potassium-rich foods. Be aware of protocols for treating hyperkalaemia.

Hypersensitivity responses	
Rash, itching, photosensitivity (increased risk of sunburn)	Report to doctor and be prepared to discontinue. Advise covering skin with clothing and high factor, high star sunscreen during exposure to direct sunlight. Avoid the midday sun in summer.
Therapeutic failure	**Pulmonary oedema not responding**: monitor vital signs regularly and maintain fluid balance records: inform medical staff if condition does not improve. Inadequate oral absorption of furosemide. Discuss possible change to bumetanide or torasemide with prescriber. **Hypertension not controlled**. Regular BP measurements until BP is within target range (<140/90mmHg). When stable, review BP and weight every 3–6 months and offer lifestyle advice. Two or more drugs are often needed to control hypertension.

Patient non-compliance: 2.8% discontinued due to adverse events in ALLHAT (2002). Explore whether this is due to effects on continence or impotence. Remind patient that, while timing can be flexible, a diuretic must be taken at some time on the day prescribed. Ensure patients understand the need for continuing administration, as abrupt discontinuation may be hazardous.

Thiazides may be ineffective in patients with renal problems. Review blood tests.

Rare adverse effects include: pancreatitis, bone marrow suppression (chapter 21)

Furosemide may affect the health of corneas being donated for transplant (Wigham & Hodson 1987).

Cautions and contra-indications:

◆ Previous **hypersensitivity responses.** People allergic to sulphonamides may be allergic to thiazides and furosemide.

◆ **Impaired kidney function.** Most thiazides are ineffective in renal failure. Contra-indicated if creatinine clearance/ GFR<30 ml/min. (BNF 2007). Furosemide has a prolonged action if renal function is impaired.

◆ **Impaired liver function.** Diuretics increase potassium and magnesium loss and may precipitate coma. An accurate history of alcohol intake is important (chapter 21).

◆ Pre-existing fluid and electrolyte imbalances (listed above) will be intensified.

◆ Addison's disease, gout, diabetes, lupus, porphyria may be exacerbated.

◆ Potassium-sparing diuretics are not recommended in severe, acute illness, renal failure or pregnancy.

◆ **Pregnancy.** Diuretics jeopardise the blood supply to the placenta. Used only under specialist supervision. Furosemide may cause respiratory problems in the neonate.

◆ **Breastfeeding.** Diuretics impair formation of breastmilk. Consult manufacturers' literature.

◆ **Non-medical use**, for example to dilute urine and hinder detection of performance-enhancing substances, is ill-advised.

25

Interactions (summary): Some drugs accentuate the adverse effects of diuretics:

◆ **Hypotension:** all anti-hypertensives, general anaesthetics, alcohol, benzo-diazepines, phenothiazines, antidepressants, nitrates, self-administered diuretics, such as caffeinated beverages (tea, coffee), dandelion or black cohosh herbal remedies

◆ **Loss of sodium:** carbamazepine, aminoglutethimide, potassium sparing diuretics, SSRIs

◆ **Loss of potassium:** digoxin, corticosteroids, bronchodilators, amphetamines, reboxetine, 'cold cures', liquorice, laxative over-use

- **Cardiac dysrhythmia** due to hypokalaemia: some anti-arrhythmics (amiodarone, quinidine, encainide, sotalol), some antipsychotics (e.g. sertindole, thioridazine), erythromycin
- Dangerously **high potassium** concentrations may occur if potassium-sparing diuretics are co-administered with: any potassium-rich food (e.g. cola drinks, citrus juices), herbal preparations or supplements, 'salt substitutes', ciclosporin, NSAIDs (non-steroidal anti-inflammatory drugs), ACE inhibitors, tacrolimus, oestrogen and progestogens.

Organ damage may occur if diuretics are combined with:

Drug	Organ affected
NSAIDs, cisplatin, cephalosporins	Kidney
Amiodarone, anti-arrhythmics	Heart
Aminoglycosides, vancomycin	Ear
Beta blockers	Pancreas, causing diabetes

Diuretics can be rendered ineffective by drugs which cause fluid retention: corticosteroids, oestrogens, NSAIDs.

All diuretics cause lithium, quinidine (or quinine) and amphetamines to accumulate, leading to adverse reactions.

Furosemide (frusemide) also reduces elimination of: gentamycin, cisplatinn, vancomycin, thophylline, cephaloridine.

Contributor

Howard Griffiths RN, BSc, MSc, PGCE (FE), RNT. Clinical Practice Tutor, School of Health Sciences, Swansea University

4 Beta blockers

Beta blockers protect the heart from the effects of stress, fright, excitement and exercise.

Actions: Beta blockers prevent adrenaline/epinephrine and noradrenaline/norepinephrine reaching their natural target sites on the beta receptors in the heart, blood vessels, liver, pancreas and bronchi. In this way, they block the actions of the sympathetic nervous system. The sympathetic nervous system controls the smooth muscle and glands of most organs by its actions on the alpha and beta receptors (glossary: adrenergic receptors).

Beta blockers stabilise the cardiovascular system and prevent increases in:

◆ heart rate.

◆ cardiac output.

◆ blood pressure (Box 4.1).

◆ activity of the renin-angiotensin-aldosterone system (see ACE inhibitors).

Therefore, the heart does less work, and needs less oxygen (Box 6.1).

Box 4.1 Overview of BP control and the actions of the four main drug groups

High blood pressure is dangerous in both the short and the long term. However, a sudden fall in BP can impair oxygen delivery to vital organs.

Blood pressure is altered by:	Cardiovascular drugs acting here:
1. Contraction or dilatation of the arterioles in the peripheral circulation, the 'peripheral resistance'.	Vasodilators (nitrates and calcium channel blockers), ACE inhibitors, diuretics.
2. Changes in cardiac output, either heart rate or stroke volume.	
(a) Heart rate	Beta blockers.
(b) Stroke volume. This depends on:	
◆ the contractile force of the heart muscle	Beta blockers.
◆ the volume of fluid in the circulation	ACE inhibitors, diuretics.
◆ the force the heart has to work against to expel blood. This is equivalent to the blood pressure in the main vessels.*	

* This is one mechanism for keeping BP at a constant level. It is disrupted in hypertension.

Indications:

◆ Angina.

◆ Myocardial infarction: both early reduction of workload and 2–3 years' prophylaxis against recurrence.

◆ Cardiac dysrhythmias (specialist care).

◆ Stabilised heart failure with specialist advice.

◆ Migraine prophylaxis.

◆ Anxiety, tremor (reduce tremor, heart rate and palpitations).

◆ Hyperthyroidism: propranolol quickly alleviates symptoms.

◆ Glaucoma (eye drops e.g. timolol).

◆ Hypertension, but only when diuretics, ACE inhibitors and calcium blockers have proved ineffective (RCP/BHS 2006) (Box 4.1). Reviews indicate that long-term use for hypertension has not reduced cardiovascular events in older people (Grossman & Messerli 2006).

Some beta blockers have limited indications, for example, soltalol and esmolol are reserved for patients with certain cardiac dysrhythmias.

Administration: A constant relationship between meals and administration of beta blockers may be advisable, particularly labetolol. For hypertension, once daily administration, in the morning, is usually adequate. To control angina, twice daily administration is often necessary. For some preparations, there is discretion regarding division of dose. Monitor any symptoms (such as chest pain) or signs (e.g. BP) before doses are due, and discuss with prescriber adjusting or increasing dose frequencies, to achieve 24 hour control. Most cardiovascular events occur between 6.00 a.m. and noon therefore it may be advisable to ensure adequate therapy at this time (Lemmer 2003).

Slow intravenous administration is undertaken with continuous monitoring.

28

Adverse effects:

◆ **Bronchospasm.** Stimulation of beta$_2$ receptors dilates the airways (see bronchodilators). Beta blockers allow the smooth muscle of the airways to contract, causing narrowing or spasm.

◆ **Cardiovascular depression.** When heart failure begins, the sympathetic nervous system compensates, but beta blockers blunt this response. Although beta blockers are prescribed for patients with heart failure, they may reduce the ability of the heart to expel blood, and thereby increase congestion. Low cardiac output may affect other systems.

◆ **Peripheral vasoconstriction.** Blood supply to muscle depends on the beta$_2$ receptors, particularly in cold environments and on exercise. Patients taking beta blockers cannot increase blood supply to muscles or raise metabolic rate on exercise or exposure to cold.

◆ **Hypoglycaemia.** Beta receptors play an important role in increasing the output of glucose from the liver during fasting. Beta blockers impair this response, and can lower blood sugar.

- ◆ Hypoglycaemia is a physiological stress, which stimulates release of adrenaline, causing sweating, tremor, tachycardia and nervousness (see insulin). Beta blockers abolish this response.
- ◆ **Changes in metabolism.** The SNS increases metabolic rate in response to the cold and exercise. This entails using glucose and lipids (fats) from the circulation. For glucose and lipids to be taken into cells, increased insulin secretion is needed. This is achieved as adrenaline stimulates the beta$_2$ receptors in the pancreas to release insulin, but is blocked by long-term beta blockers. Therefore, the concentrations of lipids and glucose in the circulation rise.
- ◆ CNS effects (below)
- ◆ **Gastrointestinal disturbances.** The GI tract is controlled by the autonomic nervous system. Beta blockers can disrupt this control, but problems are rarely serious.

Adverse effects: implications for practice: The adverse effect profile of all beta blockers is similar, including those administered as eye drops (Aronson 2006).

Potential Problem	Suggestions for Prevention and Management
Bronchospasm	
Breathing difficulties (occasionally fatal)	Check patient and family history for episodes of bronchospasm or asthma (however long ago) or respiratory conditions. Seek advice before administering if history is positive.
	Check lung function before and during therapy by peak flow or spirometry. Seek urgent review if worsening.
	In an emergency, high doses of salbutamol may be needed to reverse bronchospasm.
Cardiovascular system	
Bradycardia and possible heart block **This may reduce the blood supply to the heart muscle and cause angina**	Monitor resting heart rate. Teach patient to monitor heart rate. If <50–55 bpm, contact prescriber as dose may need to be decreased. Ensure atropine is available during intravenous administration. If heart block is suspected, ECG will be needed (see antipsychotics).
Hypotension/postural hypotension	See diuretics for patient advice and monitoring. Ensure the anaesthetic team is aware of medication prior to surgery.
Heart failure **Symptoms and signs of heart failure may be worsened or emerge:** **shortness of breath** **sleeping difficulties**	Ensure a careful record of symptoms is available. Close monitoring on initiation. Ask patients to report: ◆ breathing difficulties. ◆ any increase in the number of pillows used for sleeping.

pulmonary oedema oedema exercise intolerance loss of appetite	◆ difficulty completing sentences. ◆ any sudden weight gain or tightness of clothing or footwear. ◆ any swelling of fingers or lower legs. ◆ difficulties climbing stairs. Record patient's weight pre-therapy and every 3–6 months. Be prepared to increase the dose of diuretic and/or ACE inhibitor to balance increased fluid retention.
Reduced renal blood supply	Pre-therapy and annual test for renal function are advised for all patients with cardiovascular conditions.
Impotence/erectile dysfunction	Discuss with same-gender nurse (see diuretics).

Peripheral vasoconstriction and reduced metabolic rate

Legs become very cold Skin damage Rashes	In patients with peripheral vascular disease, observe feet and toes for any ischaemic changes. Monitor frequency of claudication (may worsen). Maintain a warm environment.
Reduced exercise tolerance/capacity, due to reduced: cardiac output, blood flow, and muscle contractility	Exercise is an important component of management of cardiovascular risk. Ask patients to monitor their physical exercise and discuss any changes with the multidisciplinary team.

Hypoglycaemia

Hypoglycaemia on fasting, particular care in children taking methylphenidate	Warn patients that severe exercise or prolonged fasting can lead to loss of consciousness due to hypoglycaemia. Discuss suitability of beta blockers for athletic and physically active patients. Monitor glucose concentrations in patients receiving dialysis.
Impaired recovery from hypoglycaemia	If diabetic patients are prescribed beta blockers, they should monitor frequency and duration of any hypoglycaemic episodes. Diabetic patients must learn to recognise hypoglycaemic episodes without relying on the characteristic rise in heart rate as a warning sign.

Changes in metabolism

Hyperglycaemia Diabetes developed in 799/9618 (8%) patients taking atenolol & 567/9639 (6%) taking amlodipine for 5.5 years, a significant difference (Dahlof *et al.* 2005)	Monitor blood glucose pre-therapy and regularly with long-term therapy (see diuretics).

Altered lipid profile (increase in triglycerides and decrease in high density lipoproteins (HDLs)). Effects may vary with different beta blockers	Monitor plasma lipids. If abnormalities arise, discuss alternative therapy. Dietary lowering of cholesterol may be less effective with beta blocker therapy.
Weight gain (1–3.5kg) due to reduced energy expenditure	Monitor body weight during first few months and long term. Seek medication review for patients trying to lose weight (Sharma *et al.* 2001).

Gastrointestinal disturbances

Dry mouth Constipation or diarrhoea Nausea	Sips of water or ice cubes may help. Attention to dental hygiene is important. Maintain fluid intake, high fibre diet and moderate exercise, if possible. Monitor bowel movements. Small frequent meals may help.

CNS effects, blunting of the SNS

Fatigue particularly on exertion Quality of life may be impaired Cognitive impairment in the elderly	Advise patients to be aware that driving may be affected, particularly in the first 3 weeks, and this will be intensified by alcohol. Report changes in mental functioning to prescriber.
Nightmares/sleep disturbance/insomnia	Patients sometimes benefit from being told that their medication is the likely cause. Changing beta blocker, to one less likely to cross the blood/brain barrier (such as atenolol), may help.
Depression, lethargy Older reviews linked beta blockers to depression	Discuss with prescriber. Advise against sudden discontinuation of medication (below).

Hypersensitivity

Anaphylaxis + failure to respond to adrenaline (rare) chapter 21 Increased risk of penicillin-induced anaphylaxis	Should anaphylaxis occur, summon urgent expert assistance. Be prepared to administer intravenous salbutamol or glucagon. Ensure a 'rescue' antihypertensive is available, for example phentolamine, nifedipine.

Withdrawal reaction

Abrupt withdrawal can lead to angina, myocardial infarction, stroke (usually occurs 2–14 days later)	Advise patients never to suddenly stop their medication. Withdrawal should be supervised gradually over several weeks. Maintain a low dose for 2 further weeks. Exercise should be restricted during this time.

Palpitations, tachycardia, sweating and tremor are relatively common	
Therapeutic failure	Advise that 2 or more drugs are often needed to reduce BP (see diuretics). Advise patients that beta blockers are less effective (or ineffective) in people who smoke tobacco. Drinking large quantities of tea or coffee has a similar, but lesser, effect.

Rare adverse effects include: hypersensitivity responses, vasculitis, migraine, psychosis, carpal tunnel syndrome, myasthenia gravis, liver disorders, tingling sensations, cramps, hair loss, and worsening of psoriasis. Vision disturbance or dry eyes should be reported.

Cautions and contra-indications:

◆ **Any history of asthma, obstructive airways disease or bronchospasm.** Relatively cardioselective drugs such as atenolol, nebivolol, betaxolol, and metoprolol have less effect on the airways and may be used cautiously by specialists.

◆ **Untreated/unstable heart failure** may be dangerously worsened. Careful monitoring is essential.

◆ Second/third degree **heart block** are contra-indications. Cautious use in first degree heart block.

◆ **Diabetes.** Betablockers are unsuitable for patients with frequent episodes of hypoglycaemia.

◆ Patients with hyperthyroidism require thyroid function tests, as clinical signs may be masked by beta blockers.

◆ Peripheral (including gastrointestinal) vascular disease, Raynaud's phenomenon, psoriasis, myasthenia gravis may worsen.

◆ Seek alternatives to beta blockers for patients at increased risk of anaphylaxis, e.g. those allergic to peanuts, if possible.

◆ Phaeochromocytoma (glossary).

◆ Decreased liver or kidney function, often necessitating lower doses.

◆ Patients receiving dialysis may be vulnerable to increased serum potassium concentrations.

◆ Sotalol (see BNF).

◆ Previous hypersensitivity to drug.

◆ **Pregnancy.** Beta blockers may cause intra-uterine growth retardation. Use in mild/moderate hypertension is rarely justified. Labetalol is prescribed in severe hypertension, with careful fetal and neonatal monitoring.

◆ **Breastfeeding.** Beta blockers pass into breastmilk, in small amounts. Some manufacturers advise to avoid.

Interactions (summary):

Hypotension is accentuated by: all anti-hypertensives, diuretics, alcohol, anti-psychotics, anti-depressants, anxioloytics/hypnotics, baclofen, vasodilators, clonidine, levodopa, anaesthetics, cimetidine.

Bradycardia is likely with co-administration of: digoxin, amiodarone, mefloquine (an anti-malarial), other anti-arrhythmics, tropisetron (an anti-emetic).

Heart failure may be precipitated by verapamil, diltiazem.

Increased vasoconstriction occurs with ergot derivatives (including ergometrine, LSD).

Hypertension may occur with co-administration of dobutamine, adrenaline (including co-administration with local anaesthetics), noradrenaline.

Impaired anti-hypertensive effects with:

◆ Drugs which stimulate the sympathetic nervous system, such as cocaine, amphetamines, cold cures containing ephedrine or pseudoephedrine, tobacco, caffeine. Salbutamol and terbutaline may act similarly.

◆ corticosteroids, oestrogens.

◆ NSAIDs (particularly piroxicam).

◆ carbamazepine, rifampicin.

Diabetes is more likely if beta blockers and diuretics, particularly thiazides, are co-prescribed long term (NICE 2006a).

Contributor
John Knight BSc, PhD. Lecturer, School of Health Sciences, Swansea University

5 Angiotensin-Converting Enzyme (ACE) Inhibitors and Angiotensin Receptor Blockers

ACE inhibitors reduce the strain on the cardiovascular system. They include captopril, enalapril, lisinopril, ramipril, cilazapril, perindopril, quinapril.

Actions: ACE inhibitors disrupt the renin-angiotensin-aldosterone system. This controls blood pressure and fluid balance (Box 4.1). ACE inhibitors block the formation of angiotensin II by the angiotensin converting enzyme, which is present in lungs, blood vessels and tissues. Angiotensin II is associated with the stress response. Its actions include constriction of blood vessels and release of aldosterone. Aldosterone allows the body to conserve sodium and water, while excreting potassium. ACE inhibitors:

◆ Reduce fluid retention and relieve heart failure by:
  ❖ increasing salt and water loss
  ❖ decreasing fluid retention and volume of fluid in the circulation
  ❖ increasing effectiveness of a failing heart
  ❖ decreasing sensation of thirst
  ❖ restoring appetite in cachexic patients (possibly).
◆ Lower BP by relaxing and dilating blood vessels (Box 4.1).
◆ Reduce arterial and myocardial stiffness, which may protect against atherosclerosis.
◆ Alter the blood flow to the kidneys (below).
◆ Disrupt the mechanisms which maintain BP on standing.
◆ Protect the linings of blood vessels, particularly in diabetes.

ACE inhibitors also prevent breakdown of inflammatory mediators, particularly the 'kinins'. Accumulation of these substances is responsible for drug-induced cough and other 'allergic-type' adverse effects.

Angiotensin-II receptor blockers/antagonists (ARBs) include losartan, irbesartan, valsartan, candesartan. Their therapeutic effects are similar to ACE inhibitors. However, they block the action (rather than formation) of angiotensin II. Their main role is control of hypertension in patients who have responded to ACE inhibitors, but who are unduly troubled by drug-induced cough.

Indications:

◆ **Heart failure or impaired left ventricular contraction** (even if there are no symptoms (Jackson 2006b)). ACE inhibitors are prescribed preferentially in the treatment of moderate-severe heart failure. Diuretics are usually co-prescribed.

◆ **Hypertension**. ACE inhibitors are first choice therapy for Caucasians (whites) under 55 years, patients with heart failure or kidney damage due to diabetes (BNF 2007), and all patients with diabetes (JSC 2006). Otherwise, they are prescribed if other treatments are not tolerated, contra-indicated or fail to control blood pressure.

◆ **Diabetic nephropathy**/ kidney disease. ACE inhibitors reduce deterioration in renal function in patients with proteinuria or microalbuminuria.

◆ **Renal disease** with proteinuria, under specialist supervision (JSC 2006). Lipid profiles may improve.

◆ **Prevention of cardiovascular events:**

  ❖ Following myocardial infarction. ACE inhibitors may be commenced within 24 hours, provided systolic BP >100mmHg and the patient is stable. Initial dose depends on systolic BP. Administration is either for 5–6 weeks or, if the left ventricle is under-performing, indefinitely.

  ❖ Stable coronary heart disease, other cardiovascular disease. The number of cardiovascular events may be reduced by 17.8% in those >55 with cardiovascular risk factors (651/4645 taking ramipril and 826/4652 taking placebo) (Yusuf *et al.* 2000).

Administration: ACE inhibitors should be taken at the same time each day, with consistent relation to meals, as absorption may be affected by food, particularly valsartan. Morning administration may be advised, to avoid excessive fall in BP at night (Lemmer 2003). Therapy is initiated with low doses, and gradual increments. Doses are adjusted at 2–4 week intervals in relation to BP and assessed immediately before a dose is due.

Adverse effects:

◆ **Hypotension.** Marked lowering of BP may occur in patients who have high concentrations of the hormone renin, which controls BP (*via* angiotensin II and aldosterone, above). This occurs when renin rises to maintain BP in response to salt depletion (e.g. diuretic use), dehydration and poor renal circulation (e.g. heart failure, vasodilator therapy). ACE inhibitors blunt the effectiveness of these responses. If the patient has been depending on renin to maintain an adequate BP, administration of ACE inhibitors can cause a sudden fall in BP, particularly on standing.

◆ **Deterioration in renal function.** When blood flow to the kidneys is poor (e.g. if the blood vessels are narrowed by atheroscleroasis) Angiotensin II maintains glomerular filtration rate (GFR). Without angiotensin II, GFR falls, and wastes, such as creatinine, accumulate (chapter 21). When the blood supply to the kidney is good, this does not happen, and ACE inhibitors do not impair renal function.

◆ **Electrolyte imbalance.** ACE inhibitors reduce the **secretion of aldosterone**. This hormone is responsible for saving salt/sodium from the distal tubule (Figure 3.1) in exchange for potassium. Without aldosterone, as sodium is lost, potassium may accumulate.

◆ **Hypersensitivity/'allergic' responses** are caused by accumulation of kinins. These cause irritation and fluid retention in mucous membranes and the skin, which reverses on discontinuation.

◆ Also: gastrointestinal and neurological effects.

Adverse effects: implications for practice: ACE INHIBITORS

Potential Problem	Suggestions for Prevention and Management
Hypotension	
Profound first dose hypotension, particularly patients taking diuretics or antihypertensives **Patients with previous myocardial infarction or stroke are at risk of recurrence if BP falls too much.**	If possible, prescriber may withdraw or reduce diuretics 2–3 days before initiation. Monitor cardiovascular condition prior to administration, and following first dose. (See cautions). If patient becomes dizzy or hypotensive, place in a supine position, offer oral fluids, and inform prescriber urgently. Ensure intravenous fluids are available. Ensure atropine is available, should heart rate fall. Following myocardial infarction, withhold and contact prescriber if systolic BP <90mmHg for >1 hour.
Hypotension/postural hypotension **4.2%, (n = 2289) patients with heart failure discontinued candesartan due to hypotension (Young et al. 2004)**	Monitor postural hypotension and advise appropriately (see diuretics). Hypotension should be reported to prescriber, and therapy reduced. Ask patients to: ◆ report any dizziness. ◆ avoid fluid depletion/ maintain fluid intake. ◆ ensure prompt rehydration during vomiting, diarrhoea or sweating. Prior to surgery, including emergency procedures, inform anaesthetic team that ACE inhibitors have been administered.
Deterioration in renal function	
Potential for kidney damage (chapter 21) **Problems are most likely in patients with heart failure, peripheral vascular disease, dehydration, diuretic therapy**	Explain that prompt recognition is essential, because timely cessation of therapy often reverses deterioration. Measure concentrations of creatinine and potassium in venous blood samples and protein in urine: ◆ pre-therapy. ◆ 1–2 weeks after initiation or dose increase ◆ during illness. ◆ during dehydration. ◆ at least annually. Refer to specialist if creatinine >150micromol/l. Following myocardial infarction, serum creatinine >177micromol/l and proteinuria >500mg/24 hours preclude therapy (ABPI 2007 Zestril® data sheet). Obtain value for GFR (chapter 21).

Electrolyte imbalance	
Hyperkalaemia **Particular caution if renal function is poor**	Monitor potassium concentrations. If >8mmol/l, there is a risk of a sudden cardiac event: inform prescriber urgently. Avoid concurrent administration of drugs increasing serum potassium (see interactions), including non-prescription products. Caution against regular self-medication with NSAIDs. Advise patient to avoid excessive consumption of potassium-rich foods e.g. bananas.
Hyponatraemia (rare)	Values for sodium concentrations are available alongside potassium.
Hypersensitivity responses	
Persistent dry cough, affecting 5–30% taking ACE inhibitors, 3–4% taking ARBs, particularly women and Chinese patients **This may arise at any dose, any time during therapy**	For hypertensive patients, co-prescription of nifedipine may ameliorate symptoms and allow dose reduction. Advise that cough may spontaneously remit and will disappear about four days after discontinuation of therapy. Advise minimising other irritants, such as chilli pepper (Fugh-Berman 2000). Suggestions include: ◆ sodium cromoglycate inhalations. ◆ low dose aspirin (interactions, below). ◆ iron supplements, but FBC must be checked first. ◆ switching to an ARB. Changing to an alternative ACE inhibitor is unlikely to help (Aronson 2006, Jackson 2006b).
Sinusitis, rhinitis	Ensure symptoms are not due to infection. Manage symptoms conservatively (as above).
Skin rash (1–2%), sometimes associated with pruritus, urticaria, photosensitivity (sunburn), hair loss **Psoriasis may be worsened**	Inform prescriber. Mild symptoms may respond to dose reduction, emollients or brief course of antihistamines. Advise covering skin with clothing and sunscreen during exposure to direct sunlight. Withhold drug and seek urgent medical opinion if severe symptoms occur.
Angioedema of nose, throat, mouth, larynx, lips and tongue, affecting 0.1–0.2% of patients within first few hours or days of therapy **Recurrent facial or tongue swelling**	Withhold drug and seek urgent medical opinion. Ensure patient is observed, as swelling may progress to airway. Ensure airway remains patent. If airway is involved, adrenaline/epinephrine, oxygen, anti-histamines, corticosteroids and intubation may be necessary. If swelling is confined to the face, anti-histamine treatment may be prescribed. Place a warning on the patient's notes, to prevent further administration.

Severe abdominal pain due to angioedema of gut, usually 1–2 days after initiation or dose change	Be aware that this may be medication-related.
Leucopenia (low white cell count)	Ask patients to report infections, e.g. sore throat, fever, as these may indicate serious adverse reactions. Obtain full blood count (FBC) to evaluate these symptoms. Obtain regular FBCs in patients with collagen vascular diseases, such as systemic lupus.
Anaemia (particularly patients with transplants), and other blood disorders (rare)	FBC is routinely checked in patients with heart failure and hypertension.

Gastrointestinal side effects

Indigestion Nausea, vomiting Diarrhoea Constipation	Advise regular meals. Ensure prompt rehydration, as fluid depletion may cause hypotension. Advise regarding constipation (see vasodilators).
Alteration or loss of sense of taste (particularly captopril)	Reassure that this common problem reverses on cessation of treatment. Encourage good mouth care/dental hygiene. Monitor diet and weight in the elderly.
Altered liver function Cholestatic jaundice Hepatitis Pancreatitis (rare)	Report severe abdominal pain and emesis urgently, withdrawal of therapy may be necessary.

Neurological side effects (relatively common)

Headache Dizziness, fatigue, malaise, insomnia, parasthesia, myalgia, mood changes, blurred vision	Paracetamol may be recommended for headache. Advise patients to ensure they are not adversely affected before driving.
Impotence	Discuss quality of life and compliance with same-gender nurse. Alternative antihyperensives are unlikely to help.

Therapeutic failure

Hypertension frequently requires 2 or 3 drugs Cardiovascular disease is likely to progress	Regularly assess presenting clinical problem. Advise patient against: ◆ high salt intake. Reduce to 2.4g sodium/day.

◆ smoking.
◆ co-administration of NSAIDs.

Co-administration with antacids reduces absorption: separate administration by 2 hours.

Be prepared to refer to prescriber: monotherapy is frequently ineffective in hypertension, and a low dose of a diuretic is usually needed (Aronson 2006).

Rare but serious adverse effects include: reduced white cell count/bone marrow suppression, epidermal necrolysis, vasculitis, fever (chapter 21).

Cautions and contra-indications:

◆ **Heart failure.** ACE inhibitors should be initiated under specialist supervision (manufacturers advise in hospital) if patients are receiving multiple or high-dose diuretic therapy (equivalent to 80mg frusemide daily), or high-dose vasodilator therapy or have:
   ❖ severe or unstable heart failure
   ❖ hypovolaemia/ dehydration
   ❖ serum sodium concentration <130 mmol/litre;
   ❖ systolic blood pressure <90mmHg;
   ❖ creatinine concentration >150 micromol/litre;
   ❖ age >70 (BNF 2007).

◆ Poor blood flow in the kidneys (**renovascular disease**) may be worsened. Without pre-therapy checks of renal function (chapter 21), this may go undiagnosed.

◆ Bilateral **renal artery stenosis.** ACE inhibitors reduce or abolish urine formation, causing severe, progressive renal failure.

◆ **Impaired renal function** hinders elimination of ACE inhibitors. Lower doses are prescribed under specialist supervision (BNF appendix 3).

◆ **Previous hypersensitivity response** to any ACE inhibitor, other forms of angioedema. Risk of angioedema very high.

◆ **Conditions reducing cardiac output,** such as aortic stenosis, cardiomyopathy. Risk of hypotension very high.

◆ **Dialysis.** Additional precautions are detailed by manufactureres.

◆ **Pregnancy.** ACE inhibitors are contra-indicated, as they can damage fetal kidneys and cause growth defects. Damage occurs *after* the first trimester (Jackson 2006b).

◆ **Breastfeeding.** ACE inhibitors pass into breastmilk. Manufacturers advise to avoid.

39

Interactions (summary):

Increased risk of hyperkalaemia with: heparins, beta blockers, NSAIDs, ciclosporin, potassium-sparing diuretics, potassium salts.

Hypotension is accentuated by: all anti-hypertensives, diuretics, alcohol, alpha-blockers, anti-psychotics, anxioloytics/hypnotics, baclofen, beta blockers, vasodilators, clonidine, levodopa, anti-depressants.

Antagonism of anti-hypertensive effect by: corticosteroids, oestrogens. NSAIDs not only antagonise the hypotensive effects, but also increase risks of kidney damage.

◆ Low dose aspirin may be co-prescribed to reduce risks of cardiovascular events. Not known to clinically reduce the efficacy of ACE inhibitors.

◆ High dose aspirin (>300mg/day) may reduce antihypertensive efficacy of ACE inhibitors by up to 50% (BNF 2007).

Ciclosporin with ACE inhibitors can result in acute kidney failure or a more gradual accumulation of potassium.

Hypoglycaemic effects of insulin, metformin and sulphonylureas are enhanced. While this is likely to be beneficial, blood glucose monitoring is needed.
Lithium, digoxin, allopurinol, procainamide are likely to accumulate.

Desensitisation treatments should not be undertaken concurrently, due to risks of anaphylaxis.

Contributor
David Gallimore BSc, MSc, RGN. Tutor in Adult Nursing, School of Health Sciences, University of Wales, Swansea

6 Vasodilators: Calcium Channel Blockers and Nitrates

Vasodilators 'open up' the circulation, easing the work of the heart, and reducing its oxygen demands (Box 6.1).

Actions: Vasodilators increase the diameter of arterioles (small muscular arteries) and veins by relaxing the smooth muscle in their walls. Vasodilatation reduces BP (Box 4.1).

Calcium channel blockers reduce movement of calcium ions into muscle cells in the heart, blood vessels and other smooth muscle. With fewer calcium ions, muscle cells contract less well.

Calcium channel blockers may:

◆ Relax arterioles. This widening of the vessels reduces the resistance to blood flow; therefore, the heart does less work while pumping blood, and needs less oxygen. (Box 6.1.)

◆ Slow the heart rate.

◆ Delay cardiac conduction.

Nitrates release nitric oxide. This is an important signalling chemical, which relaxes smooth muscle in blood vessels, airways, gut and genito-urinary tract. Nitrates:

◆ Increase the diameter of veins, which reduces the volume of blood returning to the heart. Therefore, the heart has less blood to pump out, and will do less work and need less oxygen. (Box 6.1.)

◆ Relieve acute chest pain by (Rang *et al.* 2007):

❖ relieving spasm of: coronary arteries, oesophagus and/or biliary tract

❖ opening the collateral circulation in the heart, thus bypassing diseased vessels.

◆ Relieve biliary or oesophageal spasm, which may be mistaken for angina.

Box 6.1 Oxygen and the heart

The heart needs a constant supply of oxygen for energy to pump blood around the body. The work, and oxygen, needed to do this depends on many factors. Problems arise if the heart needs more oxygen than it receives. If oxygen demand exceeds oxygen supply, the patient experiences:

◆ chest pain or

◆ arrhythmia dysrhythmia or

◆ heart failure.

Factors affecting the balance between the myocardium's oxygen supply and demand can be summarised:

	Increased by:	Decreased by:
Oxygen needs of heart muscle	Raised heart rate Hypertension Stress Anxiety Exercise	Controlling heart rate and BP Relaxation
	Drugs Adrenaline and similar drugs (e.g. amphetamines, cocaine, beta$_2$ agonists) that raise heart rate Antimuscarinics (including many antipsychotics, some anti-emetics) that raise heart rate Thyroid hormones	Beta blockers (lower heart rate) Morphine or diamorphine given intravenously
Oxygen supply to heart muscle	Being fit Oxygen administration	Poor lung function, poor cardiovascular function, for example in shock (glossary) Narrow coronary arteries Anaemia (severe)
	Drugs Vasodilators	Vasoconstrictors: cocaine, amphetamines, tobacco, cannabis, LSD, triptans, prescribed for migraine (occasionally) (El Menyar 2006, BNF 2007)

Indications and administration (summary):

Calcium channel blockers

◆ **Verapamil** acts on the heart. It is only indicated for cardiac dysrhythmias, angina and hypertension. Because verapamil reduces cardiac contractions, it is never prescribed for patients with any degree of heart failure or conduction impairment.

◆ **Nifedipine**, nicardipine, and amlodipine act on blood vessels. They are indicated in hypertension (particularly in patients with airways disease, but rarely as sole therapy (NICE 2006a)), stable angina, Raynaud's phenomenon (nifedipine only). Nifedipine is only recommended for long-term therapy in modified, slow-release forms. Dose varies with brand. Brands are not bioequivalent (glossary) and therefore not interchangeable. Nifedipine is used in premature labour (unlicensed).

◆ **Diltiazem** acts on both heart and blood vessels. Dose depends on formulation.

Tablets are swallowed whole with water, on a full stomach. Patients should be told that the outer membrane of some slow-release preparations may appear in stools.

Nitrates

Nitrates are prescribed in three forms:

	Onset of action	Duration
Glyceryl trinitrate	1 minute	20–30 minutes
Isosorbide dinitrate	<6 minutes	Up to 12 hours as slow-release
Isosorbide mononitrate	1 hour	At least 12 hours as slow-release

Some nitrates need to be stored away from light, moisture and temperature extremes. Nitrate infusions may interact with PVC containers; glass or polyethylene containers are used (ABPI 2007). Gloves should be worn when handling nitrates, to prevent absorption through the skin.

Acute attacks of angina

Glyceryl trinitrate (GTN), for example, as aerosol spray (1–2 spray doses) or sublingual tablet(s). Advise patients that these may cause a burning sensation. Frequent use (>twice/week) requires review of therapy. A spray may work more rapidly than tablets.
   Dentures and dry mouth may interfere with absorption (see interactions, below).

Angina prophylaxis

GTN, for example, as buccal tablets. Rotate sites to prevent dental caries.
   GTN patches (dose varies with brand) and ointments: dose titration requires careful observation and reporting to prescriber. Patches are sometimes used in cancer pain (Aronson 2006) (Box 13.1).

Heart Failure (adjunct)

Tablets, for example isosorbide dinitrate, isosorbide mononitrate. Injections and infusions e.g. isosorbide dinitrate 2–20mg/hour. Avoid contact with PVC.

Maintain venous patency for intravenous cannulae

GTN transdermal patches 5mg/24 hours (certain brands licensed).

Adverse effects:

ALL VASODILATORS:

- **Excessive vasodilatation:**
  - ❖ Dilatation of blood vessels causes flushing or swelling/oedema.
  - ❖ As blood vessels within the confined space of the skull dilate, intra-cranial pressure rises, causing headache.
  - ❖ Dilated blood vessels lose more heat from the body, and thermoregulatory mechanisms may not be able to compensate.
- **Hypotension.** (consequence of vasodilatation). The blood supply to the heart depends on BP remaining above a critical level, so that there is sufficient pressure to force the blood into the coronary arteries. Below this level, the heart becomes short of oxygen, and chest pain occurs. In the older people, low BP may reduce cerebral blood flow, impairing functioning of the brain.
- **Heart rate changes.** As BP falls, the SNS raises the heart rate to compensate by increasing cardiac output. (This is the baro-receptor reflex.) However, drugs may have a separate effect on the heart's pacemakers, slowing the heart rate. Therefore, the change in heart rate cannot be predicted for any one individual.

Adverse effects: implications for practice: VASODILATORS

The common adverse effects of nitrates and calcium channel blockers are similar and relate to vasodilation. Calcium channel blockers have other adverse effects, related to their action on cell membranes throughout the body.

44

Potential Problem	Suggestions for Prevention and Management
All vasodilators	
Vasodilation	
Headaches and flushing	Be prepared to administer paracetamol.
	Reassure patient this is a normal reaction.
	Administration with food may alleviate the problem with calcium channel blockers.
	Advise patients to anticipate this problem some 30–60 minutes after oral administration (Michel 2006).
	If problem intensifies during first few weeks of therapy, discuss with prescriber the possibility of increasing duration of action and the need to review regimen.
	For patients taking once daily modified release nitrate preparations, consider, with prescriber, if more frequent dosing may be less troublesome in the early stages of therapy.
Oedema – mainly calcium channel blockers	Monitor weight (see diuretics).
	Examine lower legs for oedema, skin changes and skin breakdown.
	When sitting, elevate legs.

	A daily/afternoon rest in a horizontal position may help. Encourage regular activity. Minimise salt intake (to 2.4g/day). Monitor for signs of heart failure with all calcium channel blockers (below).
Hypothermia	Maintain warm and comfortable environment.
Hypotension, orthostatic hypotension, dizziness, nausea, sweating, pallor, weakness, even fainting **Particularly if patients have Parkinson's disease**	Administer injections slowly. Maintain adequate fluid intake. Record BP before therapy and regularly thereafter. Seek advice before administration if systolic BP<90mmHg. Measure BP lying/sitting and standing: a fall in systolic BP >20mmHg or 10% indicates orthostatic hypotension (see diuretics). Assess carefully before mobilising. Change position slowly. Avoid prolonged standing, hot showers, exposure to hot environment. Avoid constipation to prevent straining during defecation (see laxatives). Advise that driving may be affected, particularly on starting treatment. Warn patients that this response is accentuated by alcohol. Advise patients that problems are usually alleviated by lying down, and elevating legs, if necessary. Discuss dose reduction with prescriber.
Worsening angina, particularly in the elderly (BP falls so low that coronary perfusion falls, reducing oxygen delivery to heart muscle)	Note relation to medication administration and report. Check for hypotension while patient is symptomatic, if possible.
Alteration in heart rate (bradycardia or tachycardia)	Check pulse before administration. If <60 or >100 consult prescriber. Administration with food may ameliorate a tachycardia.
Impaired cognitive function reported with nitrates	Review of mental state pre-therapy and regularly for older patients with impaired cognition (Aronson 2006).
Hypersensitivity responses	
Rashes, hair loss **Bronchospasm with calcium channel blockers (rare)**	Report to prescriber. Prepare to discontinue medication: an itching rash may indicate a serious reaction. Review GTN ointment: the excipient wool fat can cause rashes.

45

Withdrawal	
Exacerbation of angina or heart attack within a few days of abrupt withdrawal of regular therapy	Discuss adherence to therapeutic regimen. Inform patient of consequences of sudden withdrawal. Gradual reduction of dose prior to withdrawal.

ADDITIONAL ADVERSE EFFECTS: IMPLICATIONS FOR PRACTICE: CALCIUM CHANNEL BLOCKERS:

◆ **Gastrointestinal disturbances.** Like other muscle, the smooth muscle of the GI tract needs calcium ions to contract. Calcium channel blockers interfere with calcium ion uptake; therefore, the gut is less able to contract. GI stasis may affect the:
  ❖ lower oesophagus, causing reflux
  ❖ stomach causing nausea
  ❖ colon causing constipation.

◆ **Worsening heart failure.** Calcium ions are important for the contraction of all muscle, including heart muscle. Therefore, calcium channel blockade (particularly verapamil) can reduce the force of contraction of heart muscle, weakening the heart and impairing its ability to pump blood. Any reduction in cardiac output may precipitate heart failure in those with impaired cardiac function, such as older people (Aronson 2006). In addition, dilation of the pulmonary blood vessels can allow fluid to accumulate in the lungs. Studies report different effects of long-term calcium channel blockers on cardiovascular disease (Maxwell *et al*. 2000, Brown *et al*. 2000, Poole-Wilson *et al*. 2004).

◆ **Nervous/endocrine systems.** Many cells of the body depend on calcium ion entry to function. Occasionally, disruption of this process affects sensory, motor and endocrine systems.

Potential Problem	Suggestions for Prevention and Management
Gastrointestinal disturbances	
Taste changes	Taste may normalise with continued therapy.
Nausea/anorexia	Small regular meals. Monitor weight.
Heartburn	Avoid meals before lying down.
Constipation	Regular physical activity, adequate fluids (see diuretics) and diet (see laxatives).
Gastrointestinal obstruction/colicky pain	Be aware that some outer membranes from slow-release preparations can obstruct the gut.
Gingival (gum) hyperplasia is thought to be due to increased testosterone production	Scrupulous oral hygiene. Liaise with dental hygienist and dentist experienced with this condition.

GI bleeding (rare)	Report any black stools or other signs of blood loss.
Worsening heart failure	
Breathlessness, cough, wheeze, pulmonary oedema	Observe patients when talking. Inability to complete a sentence is a sign of pulmonary oedema. Monitor patients for indications of worsening heart failure (see beta blockers).
Nervous/endocrine systems	
Insomnia/fatigue **Nervousness, loss of energy, mood changes cramps/stiffness**	Encourage regular activity.
Frequency of micturition	Ensure adequate fluid intake.
Posture and movement disorders (rare) (Aronson 2006)	Be alert for abnormal movements or stiffness, which may be early signs of Parkinsonism. Refer to prescriber.
Impotence	Refer to specialist service or prescriber.

Rare adverse effects include: eye pain, menorrhagia, breast discomfort (see anti-psychotics).

 ## Additional adverse effects: NITRATES

Potential Problem	Suggestions for Prevention and Management
Therapeutic failure	
Chest pain does not respond	Check administration technique: ensure that spray is directed under tongue and mouth is closed after administration. Check buccal preparations have not been swallowed. Check position of dentures. Ensure mucous membranes are moist. Ensure GTN tablets are kept in original containers and, once opened, discarded after 8 weeks. Failure to respond to 3 doses over 15 minutes may indicate a myocardial infarction or an alternative source of pain (Michel 2006). Check oxygen saturation. Occasionally, this may fall on administration, as blood vessels in the lungs dilate. Suggest that patient keeps a diary of symptoms, including time of day. Ensure nitrates are infused from glass or polyethylene equipment.

Chest pain no longer responds	Reduce blood nitrate concentration to low levels for 4–8 hours each day by:
With repeated use, tolerance arises from changes in the enzymes of the vessel walls	◆ administering twice daily medication at 8 and 16 hour intervals. ◆ removing and not replacing patches for several consecutive hours. Choose times when angina is least frequent. Seek alternative therapy if angina rebounds during nitrate-free intervals. Time nitrate-free intervals at night, unless angina is worse at night. This is most likely in patients who sleep on several pillows.

Cautions and contra-indications:

All vasodilators

◆ Hypotension, hypovolaemia, hypothermia will be exacerbated, due to loss of effective circulating volume and loss of heat through peripheral vasodilatation.

◆ Aortic or mitral stenosis.

◆ Recent heart attack.

◆ Pulmonary hypertension.

◆ Severe hepatic or renal failure may be worsened. Careful monitoring is required.

◆ Previous hypersensitivity to the product.

Nitrates: Further contra-indications and cautions include: cardiac tamponade, constrictive pericarditis, marked anaemia, closed-angle glaucoma, hypothyroidism.

Nitrates should be given to patients with head trauma and cerebral haemorrhage only in cases where no other vasodilator is clinically suitable.

GTN transdermal patches should be removed before cardioversion or diathermy.

Calcium channel blockers: Further cautions and contra-indications include:

◆ Doses are reduced for elderly patients.

◆ Unstable angina.

◆ Heart failure, heart block or other conditions slowing the heart: verapamil, diltiazem contra-indicated. Nifedipine is used with caution (BNF 2007).

◆ Some slow-release preparations are contra-indicated in patients with risk of bowel obstruction, e.g. inflammatory bowel disease, narrowing of gastrointestinal tract, or Koch pouch (internal reservoir connecting to stoma).

◆ Pregnancy. Fetal damage has occurred in animals: manufacturers advise avoid in women of child-bearing age.

◆ Breastfeeding. These drugs enter breast milk, although the clinical significance is unclear. Manufactures advise avoid.

◆ Rarely, diabetes may be worsened.

48

Interactions (summary):

All vasodilators: Enhanced hypotension may be caused by co-administration of: any anti-hypertensive agent, alcohol, general anaesthetic, diuretic, levodopa, antipsychotics, antidepressants.

Hypotension is particularly likely if:

◆ nitrates are administered within 24 hours of sildenafil and longer with tadalafil.

◆ nifedipine is co-administered with parenteral magnesium sulphate.

◆ calcium channel blockers are combined with alpha-blockers (e.g. tamsulosin for prostatic hypertrophy), particularly on first dose.

Vasodilators are **antagonised** by: coticosteroids, NSAIDs, oestrogens.

Calcium channel blockers: Co-administration of beta blockers may cause severe hypotension, bradycardia, heart failure or, with verapamil, asystole. This problem is rarer with nifedipine and related drugs (Baxter 2006), but the interaction is marked as 'potentially hazardous' (BNF 2007, p. 696).

Hypotension is likely with: grapefruit/grapefruit juice (Dresser *et al.* 2000, 2002), cimetidine, ketoconazole, ciclosporin.

Effects of calcium channel blockers are reduced by: barbiturates, carbamazepine, phenytoin.

Calcium channel blockers potentiate: carbamazepine, ketoconazole, itraconazole, mefloquine, benzodiazepines, theophylline, immunosuppressants, amiodarone, digoxin, lithium, muscle relaxants, ciclosporin, some anti-viral agents.

49

Nitrates: Drugs reducing saliva production (tricyclic antidepressants, antimuscarinics (e.g. procyclidine), antipsychotics, lithium), smoking, eating and drinking reduce absorption of preparations absorbed through the mouth.

Intravenous GTN increases excretion of heparin, reducing the anticoagulant effect: coagulation tests must be undertaken regularly.

Contributor

David Gallimore BSc, MSc, RGN. Tutor in Adult Nursing, School of Health Sciences, University of Wales, Swansea

7 Anticoagulants

Anticoagulants reduce formation of new blood clots and extension of existing clots, particularly in veins. They do not dissolve existing clots.

Actions: Normal blood flow depends on the delicate balance between clotting and anti-clotting factors. Anticoagulants affect this balance by:

◆ immediately boosting the anti-clotting factors (heparin).

◆ interrupting the production of clotting factors, over a period of 5 days (warfarin).

Heparin occurs naturally in the body, mainly in the lungs, but also in the liver and intestines. It augments/boosts the function of the body's own naturally occurring inhibitor of coagulation, antithrombin III. This inactivates nearly all the clotting factors. Low molecular weight (LMW) heparins act on clotting factor Xa (prothrombinase); they include dalteparin, enoxaparin, tinzaparin.

Warfarin is one of the coumarin drugs. It has a similar molecular structure to vitamin K, which is involved in the synthesis of clotting factors II, VII, IX, and X and anti-clotting factors (proteins C and S) in the liver. Warfarin depletes the supply of active vitamin K, thus affecting the clotting factors necessary for coagulation. This mode of action means that warfarin takes between two and three days to have a clinical effect.

Indications include:

◆ Pulmonary emboli (PE) and deep-vein thromboses (DVT) are initially managed with heparin or LMW heparin. Warfarin is commenced simultaneously. Heparin is discontinued when results of coagulation tests permit.

◆ Prophylaxis for PE and DVT during periods of immobility, before and 7–10 days after surgery or until mobile: usually LMW heparins. Risks are high some 7–10 days after surgery.

◆ Acute management of myocardial infarction, unstable angina, arterial occlusion, extra-corporeal circulation: heparins.

◆ Long-term prophylaxis for patients with prosthetic heart valves, atrial fibrillation or myocardial infarction (in certain circumstances): usually warfarin.

◆ Heparin flushes maintain patency of cannulae. Saline is equally effective for venous cannulae.

Administration: Heparin is administered by injection, usually short term. There are two types:

◆ standard/unfractionated heparin, which acts immediately on most clotting factors

◆ low-molecular-weight (LMW) heparins, which act mainly on one clotting factor (Xa) and last up to 24 hours.

Standard heparin is administered by either continuous intravenous infusion (sometimes preceded by loading dose) or 12-hourly subcutaneous injections. Duration of action ranges from 2–6 hours, depending on dose administered. Anticoagulation diminishes rapidly when infusion is discontinued. Therefore, this form of heparin is sometimes preferred for patients at high risk of bleeding. Heparin sodium is available in three concentrations. Heparin calcium, is prescribed less frequently. Dose depends on patient's condition, weight, age and treatment response.

Low molecular weight heparins are administered by sub-cutaneous injection, from manufacturers' pre-filled syringes (usually once or twice daily) (see Figure 10.4):

◆ Explain procedure, gain informed consent.

◆ With the patient supine, identify administration site in abdominal wall (or lateral thigh for some preparations e.g. dalteparin). Site at least 5cm from umbilicus or any scars.

◆ Make a thick skin fold by squeezing the skin between the thumb and index finger. This ensures heparin is not injected into muscle.

◆ Introduce the whole length of needle into this fold, at 90° to the skin.

◆ Inject, hold for 10 seconds. Release skin only when injection is complete.

◆ Avoid rubbing.

◆ Application of ice may reduce pain, but not haematoma formation (Ross & Solters 1995).

◆ Document and rotate sites (ABPI 2007) (Figure 16.1).

Maximum effect is anticipated some 2 hours after administration, depending on preparation. Different heparins are not bioequivalent and should not be interchanged during treatment without authorisation from prescriber.

Warfarin is administered orally, once daily, at the same time, with a constant relation to food intake. Dose depends on the patient's International Normalised Ratio (INR) (glossary).

51

Adverse effects: implications for practice: All anticoagulants disable the
clotting mechanisms, increasing the risk of bleeding, particularly at high doses.

Potential Problem	Suggestions for Prevention and Management
Bleeding	
All anticoagulants **Women over 60, patients with history of bleeding, liver disease, alcoholism, vascular disease, hypertension, cancer, thyroid disease, renal disease or platelet deficiency and those who do not adhere to their therapeutic regimen are at greatest risk**	**Before and during therapy, check:** FBC (including platelets), coagulation tests, electrolytes, urine and stools for occult bleeding, BP (seek advice if uncontrolled hypertension suspected). **Monitor**: ◆ bleeding in catheter sites, drains, mouth ◆ pressure area problems ◆ symptoms of internal bleeding, e.g. low back pain ◆ patients receiving intraspinal analgesia for symptoms of intraspinal haematoma, including: midline back pain and neurological deficits (such as, bowel or bladder dysfunction, numbness, motor or sensory deficits). **Avoid** intramuscular injections, catheters, enemas, rectal thermometers, if possible. Apply pressure following any essential venepuncture.

Ask patients to:

◆ Report oozing cuts, bleeding gums, bruises, nosebleeds, joint swelling, petechiae, increased menstrual loss or post-partum bleeding.
◆ Wear medi-alert bands with anticoagulant clearly written, and show this to all doctors, dentists and pharmacists.
◆ Avoid: going 'barefoot', vigorous nose blowing or teeth cleaning.
◆ Use soft toothbrushes and electric razors.

If bleeding is suspected, withhold drug and seek urgent evaluation.

Ensure surgical and anaesthetic teams are informed of all anticoagulant therapy.

Standard heparin: acute care **Major bleeding reported in 1–5% patients receiving intravenous therapy (Majerus & Tollefsen 2006). Many events occur on the third day of therapy**	Check vital signs every 4 hours, initially. Monitor APTT (activated partial thromboplastin time), or equivalent, same time each day (or as requested by prescriber), starting 4–6 hours after infusion commences, from arm not receiving infusions. Other measures of coagulation, e.g. factor Xa, are sometimes more reliable e.g. in pregnancy. Ensure 1% **protamine** sulphate is available for slow intravenous administration, should serious bleeding occur. Dose is calculated according to coagulation tests. Protamine sulphate should be administered cautiously: large quantities are anticoagulant and anaphylaxis is possible. Particular care in patients who have received certain brands of insulin (NPH or protamine zinc insulins).
Low molecular weight heparins **Risk of major bleeding up to 3%**	APTT monitoring is ineffective. Factor Xa activity is assessed only if necessary. The anticoagulant effects are only partially reversed by protamine.
Warfarin **Major bleeding reported in 2–3% patients each year (Aronson 2006), minor bleeding 36% over 3 years (Warfarin Antiplatelet Investigators 2007)**	Monitor INR: pre-therapy, daily until stable, then regularly (minimum every 12 weeks). Risks increased if INR>4. Be aware of protocols for withholding medication and referral should results be outside the desired range, which depends on condition treated (BNF 2007). Ensure patients understand the need to attend clinics. Monitor compliance and clinic attendance: bleeding is more likely in non-attenders. Increase observation and INR testing if illness develops, particularly liver disease. Monitor weight and diet when patient attends coagulation clinics. Weight loss, malnutrition or illness may necessitate dose reduction. Ensure vitamin K_1 (oral or intravenous), and, in acute setting, clotting factors are available.

Therapeutic failure	
Failure of prophylaxis	**Acute care:** Check for DVT: measure and compare calf circumferences every 8 hours. Check for PE: dyspnoea, pulmonary oedema, cough and haemoptysis at least every 4 hours initially.
The risk of thrombosis depends on:	
1. **Rate of blood flow.** This is affected by mobility and dehydration or turbulent flow around narrow valves	Mobilise, encourage anti-embolic stockings. Ensure that the patient does not become dehydrated. If gastrointestinal upset occurs, ensure prompt rehydration and arrange coagulation checks. In **acute care** assist in turning, coughing and deep breathing every 4 hours
2. **Injury to the lining of the blood vessels**	Avoid constrictive clothing, leg stirrups. Extra vigilance in patients with atherosclerosis.
3. **The balance between clotting and anti-clotting factors**	Discourage smoking. Seek advice regarding any oestrogen therapy (Combined Oral Contraceptives, HRT). Be aware of higher risks associated with extensive tissue damage, disease, inherited conditions, high concentrations of oestrogens, as in pregnancy. Seek advice regarding screening for inherited clotting abnormalities, which may predict future risk of thromboembolism.

Rare adverse effects include: priapism, reversible hair loss (with long-term use), hepatitis, agranulocytosis (glossary).

 ## Heparin: additional adverse effects: implications for practice:

◆ **Heparin** may induce the formation of antibodies against platelets or tissues.

◆ **Hyperkalaemia** (high potassium concentration), and fluid loss may be due to stimulation of aldosterone secretion.

◆ **Heparin** binds to calcium ions, which affects bone, with long-term use.

◆ **Heparin resistance.** Heparin will be more rapidly destroyed in patients who smoke or have infection, cancer, extensive clotting or surgery. Heparin will also lose its effectiveness if antithrombin is in short supply, for example, if there is atherosclerosis, extensive clotting or liver or kidney disease (Lutomski *et al.* 1995).

◆ **Osteoporosis.** Heparin binds calcium ions, reducing the calcium available for bone maintenance.

Potential Problem	Suggestions for Prevention and Management
Heparin antibodies	
Low platelet count or 30–50% fall in platelet count **Highest risk 5–14 days after initiation, but earlier with previous exposure to heparin** **Mild form resolves on discontinuation. Severe form associated with thromboembolism**	Monitor platelets: pre-therapy, daily or regularly thereafter. Check for purpura/ bruising, petechiae in dependent areas and under BP cuff. Report any abnormalities. Highlight reaction on patient's notes, because further administration of any heparins might be dangerous.
Skin necrosis some 6–9 days after start of therapy	Continued observation of injection sites (see warfarin)
Electrolyte imbalance	
Hyperkalaemia particularly patients with renal failure, metabolic acidosis, diabetes, or receiving potassium-sparing diuretics or ACE inhibitors	Monitor potassium concentrations: pre-therapy (high-risk patients), after 7 days' therapy (all patients).
Diuresis on 2nd day (relatively common)	Warn patients that diuresis usually lasts 48 hours. Ensure facilities are available.
Osteoporosis	
Bone loss if administration >1 month e.g. during pregnancy	Review diet for fish and milk intake. Consider calcium supplements.
Hypersensitivity responses	
Rashes and itching at administration site, lacrimation, bronchospasm, chills, chest pain, angioedema, anaphylaxis	'Test doses' may be prescribed for patients with allergies. Observe for these problems whenever heparin is administered, including cannula 'flushes'. Tinzaparin contains sulphites and may precipitate asthma. Ensure reactions are clearly documented.
Injection site reactions: irritation, bruising, inflammatory nodules, skin necrosis	Seek alternative therapy at first signs of skin irritation, to avoid progression. Avoid heparin calcium in patients with renal failure.

Therapeutic or prophylaxis failure	
Heparin resistance, making therapy ineffective, or necessitating higher doses	Report any infection, fever or thrombophlebitis, as doses may need adjustment.

Heparin releases an enzyme which removes fat from plasma. Very rarely, rebound hyper-lipidaemia may occur on withdrawal.

 ## Additional adverse effects: implications for practice:
WARFARIN

Skin necrosis follows widespread thrombosis of the microvasculature, caused by reduced availability of anti-clotting factors; also cholesterol emboli and disruption of healing.

Potential Problem	Suggestions for Prevention and Management
Disruption of the blood supply:	
Skin necrosis (0.01–0.1% patients) Usually 3–5 days (range 4 hours–6 months) after initiation of therapy, particularly obese women	Ask patients to report painful red areas. Seek urgent medication review, as lesions rapidly progress. Ensure vitamin K is available. Seek advice regarding screening for associated inherited clotting abnormalities.
Discolouration of feet believed to be due to cholesterol emboli	Check toes for any discolouration.
Delayed healing of fractures may be due to haematoma formation or interference with ossification/bone formation	Ensure patients receive realistic advice regarding the expected rate of healing.
Therapeutic or prophylaxis failure	
Drug/food interactions may upset the balance between warfarin and vitamin K	Assess diet and stress importance of regular food intake. If INR is fluctuating, monitor intake of food supplements and vegetables (see interactions).
Diarrhoea causing loss of vitamin K and bleeding	Check INR following diarrhoea or administration of antibiotics.
Changes in weight or health status will necessitate change in dose	Monitor weight, diet and fluid intake when patient attends coagulation clinics. Weight loss, malnutrition, reduction in intake or illness will require dose reduction.

Non-compliance	Advise patients against abrupt discontinuation of warfarin without medical advice. Supervise gradual withdrawal over 3–4 weeks, with INR monitoring, as necessary.

Cautions and contra-indications:

◆ Both administration and non-administration can be detrimental, and decisions are often complex, for example, if patients have potential bleeding sites, such as hiatus hernia, peptic ulcer, neoplasms, retinopathy.

◆ **High risk of bleeding:** hemophilia, liver disease, oesophageal varices, recent cerebral haemorrhage, major trauma, purpura, thrombocytopenia, severe hypertension, active tuberculosis, peptic ulcer, high alcohol consumption, bacterial endocarditis, severe renal impairment (see BNF).

◆ **Recent trauma or surgery** to central nervous system, eye or ears, and retinopathy, where bleeding would be catastrophic.

◆ **Intraspinal analgesia and lumbar puncture** usually preclude therapeutic doses, but prophylactic doses may be administered cautiously.

◆ **Pregnancy.** Specialist advice essential. Heparin is usually prescribed. Warfarin is associated with fetal malformations of bone, brain and eyes, and intra-partum haemorrhage. Women of child-bearing age should seek specialist advice regarding contraception.

◆ **Breastfeeding.** Heparin does not appear in breastmilk. Manufacturers of LMW heparins advise avoid breastfeeding. Warfarin appears safe (BNF 2007); some authorities recommend weekly administration of vitamin K (Aronson 2006).

◆ **Children/neonates.** See manufacturers' literature. Neonates: avoid products containing benzyl alcohol e.g. some dalteparin preparations.

◆ Previous thrombocytopenia, skin necrosis or hypersensitivity.

◆ Heparin (including heparin flushes) **interferes with certain laboratory tests,** such as thyroid function tests, gentamicin concentrations. Information that patient is receiving heparin should be included on laboratory forms.

Interactions (summary): All anticoagulants. Bleeding is more likely when anticoagulants and antiplatelet drugs are co-administered, e.g. aspirin, salicylates, non-steroidal anti-inflammatory drugs, including topical preparations, long-term paracetamol. Combining heparin with dextrans increases risks of bleeding. Smokers may need higher doses.

Heparin is incompatible with many drugs when mixed within infusions and syringes e.g. antibiotics, opioids: separate heparin from other drug infusions. If heparin flushes are used, additional saline flushes are administered before and after medication administration.

Heparins may be antagonised by nitrates, streptokinase, vitamin C, tetracyclines, digitalis, and augmented by sibutramine (an appetite suppressant).

Warfarin's effects can be increased or decreased by change in availability of vitamin K, caused by medicines, diet, dietary supplements and enteral feeding. A small (10% or 50 microgram) change in the regular dietary intake of vitamin K may significantly alter INR (Thomson *et al.* 2000). Patients should be advised:

◆ Maintain constant intake of foods and supplements containing vitamins K and C e.g. brassicas, onions, lettuce, soya products, mango, green tea. Large quantities of ice-cream (1 litre) have been known to antagonise warfarin (Baxter 2006).

◆ Many herbal medicines and non-prescription products interact with warfarin, and are best avoided, particularly cranberry juice, anabolic steroids, danshen, dong quai, feverfew, *Ginko biloba* (promote bleeding), St. John's Wort, Ginseng (promotes clotting) (Fugh-Berman 2000, Baxter 2006).

◆ Interactions occasionally occur with: grapefruit juice, large quantities of alcohol, garlic, avocado, charcoal grilled meats, tonic water.

◆ Risk of bleeding is increased when absorption of vitamin K is impaired by mineral oils, large doses of vitamin E or oral antibiotics.

◆ Risk of clotting increased by a high fat diet.

Warfarin interacts with many prescription drugs: e.g. bleeding has occurred following influenza vaccination and emergency hormonal contraception. Usually, introduction of any additional medicines necessitates increased INR monitoring.

Contributor

Richard Lake RN, Dip.N, BSc (Hons), ATNC. Clinical Skills Tutor, School of Health Sciences, Swansea University

8 Bronchodilators: selective beta₂ adrenoceptor agonists

Selective beta$_2$ agonists, such as salbutamol, relieve bronchospasm by opening the small airways, which allows patients to breathe more easily.

Actions: Beta$_2$ adrenoceptor agonists have many of the same actions as adrenaline/epinephrine, the hormone of fright/flight/fight. To achieve this, they stimulate the beta$_2$ receptors in the lungs. This relaxes the smooth muscle in the walls of the airways and opens the airways, increasing the quantity of air and oxygen reaching the alveoli and the pulmonary blood capillaries. However, bronchodilators, like adrenaline, also stimulate other systems. (See glossary: adrenerigic receptors.)

Beta$_2$ adrenoceptor agonists relieve the immediate bronchospasm response to allergens (a type I reaction, chapter 21). However, they do not help, and, if used alone, may intensify the delayed inflammatory type III response which comes some 6–8 hours later. Therefore, co-administration of cromoglicate or inhaled corticosteroids is usually advised (Aronson 2006).

Indications:

◆ Reversible airways obstruction in asthma and chronic obstructive pulmonary disease (COPD).

◆ 10–15 minutes before unavoidable exposure to known asthma triggers, such as exercise.

◆ **Short-acting** selective beta$_2$ adrenoceptor agonists (salbutamol, terbutaline) are used as 'rescue' or 'reliever' therapy to control asthma and COPD (BTS 2005). They act within 5 minutes and last 4–6 hours. Used alone, they do not control night-time symptoms. If relief lasts <3 hours, inform prescriber. They are sometimes used in premature labour.

◆ **Long-acting** selective beta$_2$ adrenoceptor agonists (salmeterol, formoterol) are used in conjunction with inhaled corticosteroids to prevent symptom recurrence, with regular review. Salmeterol does not treat acute bronchospasm (BNF 2007).

Asthma management is informed by British Thoracic Society (BTS) guidelines (2005), summarised in current editions of the BNF. Any patient using a bronchodilator inhaler more than twice each week, or experiencing night-time symptoms more than once a week, should be administering regular preventive, anti-inflammatory medication, usually an inhaled corticosteroid.

Administration: Record all medications, with dates, on patients' records or diaries of asthma symptoms and peak flow recordings. Whenever possible, in patients of *all* ages, disease of the airways is managed by inhaled medication (Box 8.1). Spacer devices should be: cleaned once a month by washing in mild detergent, rinsing and allowing to dry in air; replaced every 6–12 months (Le Souëf 1999, BTS 2005).

> ## Box 8.1   Inhaler technique
>
> Ensure that the patient:
>
> ◆ understands that inhalation before meals will assist eating by reducing the fatigue caused by eating.
> ◆ knows the importance of keeping the aerosol away from the eyes.
> ◆ administers bronchodilator before corticosteroid.
> ◆ shakes the container several times before administration (otherwise only propellant will be delivered).
> ◆ exhales fully before administration.
> ◆ fully seals lips around mouthpiece.
> ◆ administers medication at the commencement of inhalation.
> ◆ inhales slowly and deeply.
> ◆ holds breath for at least a full 10 seconds before exhaling slowly through pursed lips.
> ◆ withholds further inhalations for at least one minute.
> ◆ rinses the mouth with water after each inhalation; this water should not be swallowed.
> ◆ waits 1–2 minutes before administering a second puff (if prescribed).
> ◆ waits 5 minutes before administering the next inhaled drug.

Aerosol inhalers may contain either hydrofluoroalkanes or chlorofluorocarbons as propellants. Hydrofluoroalkanes are superseding chlorofluorocarbons, because they are less damaging to the Earth's ozone layer. New propellants may give a different taste or feel. If inhalers or spacers are substituted or brands are changed, patients should be monitored for any change in bioavailability (glossary) and increase in side effects or decrease in efficacy (Micheletto *et al.* 2005, Hendeles *et al.* 2007). Canisters should be protected from direct sunlight. To facilitate ordering of replacements, it is useful to record the number of doses taken from each inhaler.

Nebulisers should be used in well-ventilated environments, as some drug escapes into the surroundings. Drug remaining in the nebuliser should be discarded after 24 hours. If necessary, nebulised drugs may be diluted with sterile sodium chloride solution 0.9%. Using water as the diluent may cause bronchospasm. When salbutamol is given by nebuliser, each dose is 25 times higher than the aerosol dose.

Dry powder inhalers contain higher doses (usually double) than aerosols, to account for their lower absorption. If they stimulate coughing, alternative delivery systems may be necessary.

Oral therapy, e.g. tablets and syrups, is associated with higher incidence of adverse effects.

Intravenous administration is reserved for severe illness.

Adverse effects:

◆ **Over-stimulation of cardiovascular system.** Beta$_2$ agonists are structurally similar to adrenaline which drives the cardiovascular system to increase cardiac output and facilitate exercise in 'fright, flight or fight'. This involves increasing the heart rate, pulse pressure, cardiac contractility and workload, and stimulating the rennin-angiotensin-aldosterone axis. This extra workload may over-tax the cardio-vascular systems of older people or new users with pre-existing cardiovascular disease receiving high dose nebulised or intravenous therapy (Box 6.1).

◆ **Dilation of blood vessels.** Stimulation of the beta$_2$ receptors dilates blood vessels. This is advantageous during exercise, but can be troublesome. Dilation of pulmon-ary blood vessels increases blood flow to the alveoli. If increased blood flow is not matched by increased air flow, the concentration of oxygen in the blood may be reduced (hypoxia).

◆ **Fluid and electrolyte imbalance** may be due to stimulation of the renin-angiotensin-alosterone axis (see ACE inhibitors).

◆ Metabolic:
  ❖ Beta$_2$ receptors in the liver prepare the body for exertion by increasing glucose output. If exercise does not happen, this glucose may accumulate in the circulation.
  ❖ Stimulation of the sympathetic nervous system may increase metabolic rate. Relative lack of oxygen may cause lactic acidosis.
  ❖ Lipid profile may be improved.

◆ **Neurological** disturbance; adrenaline induces similar responses.

◆ **Autonomic imbalance.** The sympathetic nervous system dries secretions and inhibits contraction of smooth muscle in the airways, gut, genito-urinary tract and uterus.

Adverse effects: implications for practice: BRONCHODILATORS

Monitoring for adverse effects is undertaken alongside lung function tests. The quantity of inhaled drug absorbed depends on lung function: adverse effects intensify if asthma or COPD improve, and decrease if they deteriorate.

Potential Problem	Suggestions for Prevention and Management
Cardiovascular system	
Tachycardia: excessive rise in heart rate is associated with myocardial ischaemia, chest pain, cardiac dysrhythmia, reduced cardiac output and pulmonary oedema (Vesalainen *et al.* 1999) Inhaled administration: 64% of adults complain of tachycardia (White & Sander 1999)	Assessment of cardiovascular system before and during therapy. This should include oxygen saturation, because cardiovascular problems are more likely if the patient is hypoxic. **Primary care.** Teach patient to monitor pulse before each dose and withhold doses if pulse too rapid, HR >110bpm. Advise client not to exceed recommended dosage. Monitor prescription of inhalers: a salbutamol inhaler should last 3 months; 2 preventer inhalers (usually corticosteroids) should usually be prescribed for each bronchodilator inhaler. **Acute care.** During administration of high doses: monitor pulse at least every 15 minutes (continuously with intravenous administration). ECG monitoring may be necessary, particularly in older people. Be aware that problems may arise despite a

Intravenous administration raises heart rate by 20–40 beats per minute (McKenry and Salerno 2003), but may also alleviate a tachycardia	normal ECG. Seek assistance if HR rises >135–140bpm. Problems can arise up to 12 hours after discontinuation of terbutaline.
Systolic hypertension	Monitor BP regularly in primary care and every 15 minutes during administration of high doses.

Dilation of blood vessels

Flushing, sweating, headache	Advise patients that these symptoms are relatively frequent.
Diastolic hypotension	Advise older clients to rise slowly after inhalation.
Hypoxia during nebulised therapy (particular danger in children <18 months)	Check oxygen saturation. For most patients, administer oxygen during nebulisation, **but avoid oxygen if the patient's carbon dioxide concentration is raised.**

Fluid and electrolyte imbalance

Fluid retention and pulmonary oedema, leading to hypoxia, during administration of high doses	Strict fluid balance records. Limit fluid intake to 2.5 litres/24 hours. Observe for shortness of breath, inability to finish sentences. Listen to lung bases with a high quality stethoscope. Avoid saline infusions. Assess body weight before and during therapy. Ensure diuretics and potassium monitoring available. Extra care if infection present.
Hypokalaemia (glossary) can cause: ◆ Cardiac dysrhythmia, even arrest ◆ Muscle weakness, impairing respiration.	Arrange venous blood samples for electrolyte assessment pre-therapy and at follow up. **Primary care:** advise clients to eat potassium-rich foods, such as bananas, raisins, oranges, meat. **Acute care:** monitor electrolytes and ECG for signs of hypokalaemia, especially if patient is hypoxic or corticosteroids are co-administered.

Metabolism

Hyperglycaemia/diabetes	**Primary care**: pre-therapy blood glucose and regular monitoring. **Acute care**: pre-therapy and 4 hourly blood glucose measurements.
Lactic acidosis in acute therapy. The associated respiratory effort may be mistaken for worsening asthma	Arrange blood gases to assist in recognition of this problem and to avoid inappropriate dosage increments.

61

Autonomic imbalance	
Gastrointestinal tract stasis, anorexia	**Primary care:** weigh clients before and during therapy. Ask about constipation. Monitor fluid, nutrient and fibre intake in older people. Small frequent meals may help. **Acute care:** be prepared for client to feel nauseous and vomit during administration of high doses.
Glaucoma (rare)	Ensure aerosol or nebuliser does not enter eyes. Particular caution if ipratropium bromide nebulisers are used concurrently.
Drying of secretions. Irritation of mouth and throat	Ensure older patients are adequately hydrated. Offer ice cubes. Rinse mouth with water after each inhalation. Encourage deep breathing exercises to prevent chest infections. Offer advice in relation to oral hygiene. Encourage patient to stop smoking. Avoid other bronchial irritants and aerosols, e.g. hairsprays.
Worsening of pre-existing prostatic hypertrophy	Direct questioning of older men. If problem is unrecognised, retention of urine may cause infection.
Central nervous system stimulation	
Insomnia, restlessness or undue fear Confusion, agitation, hallucinations and paranoia	Avoid oral therapy, particularly at night. Suggest substituting milk for caffeine-containing drinks in the evening. Monitor any difficult behaviour in children. Inquire about hallucinations and reassure. Monitor oxygen saturation in older patients. These problems may be due to **either bronchodilators or hypoxia** from underlying respiratory condition.
Hand tremor, particularly after inhalation	Advise parents that children's handwriting may deteriorate. Tolerance may develop.
Hypersensitivity (rare)	
Increased wheezing on administration (particularly formoterol or salmeterol)	This may be a hypersensitivity response to the drug or other ingredients in inhaler. Seek alternative therapy or delivery device.
Withdrawal	
Rebound of asthma symptoms on withdrawal Patients become unduly sensitive to allergens	If the patient has been symptom-free for 3 months, continuous therapy should be withdrawn gradually. Patients should always have a spare inhaler.

Therapeutic failure: Protection against bronchial reactivity may diminish with repeated use within a week (Aronson 2006). Beta receptors become desensitised to their agonists (glossary).

Symptoms deteriorate, particularly on introduction and regular use of long-acting beta$_2$ agonists	Prevention: Monitor closely. Step down therapy once control is achieved. Warn client not to over-use medication. Seek review of prescriptions for long-acting beta$_2$ agonists (Salpeter *et al*. 2006) Seek treatment review if using more than 2 inhalers/month (BTS 2005) Consider possible causes: ◆ not using steroid regularly. ◆ poor inhaler technique (Keeley 1993). ◆ change of inhaler or spacer. ◆ inhalers becoming cold and therefore delivering less medication. Check storage conditions. ◆ Products past expiry date (lose efficacy).
Signs of worsening disease, which could easily progress to an acute episode	Inform prescriber if: ◆ usual dose becomes ineffective. ◆ inhaler is being used more frequently than usual. Effectiveness may be restored by co-administration of corticosteroids.
Symptoms of asthma worsen in the premenstrual period	A diary record of symptoms and menstruation will ensure this is detected and medication review initiated. Important at onset of puberty.
Asthma fails to respond to rescue doses of salbutamol (Hancox *et al*. 1999)	Be prepared to administer a high dose of corticosteroids if an acute asthma attack occurs.

63

Cautions and contra-indications: Adreno-ceptor agonists increase the risk of adverse cardiovascular events in those most at risk, including patients with:

◆ Pre-existing risk factors for cardiac disease and myocardial hypoxia:
  ❖ angina
  ❖ hypertension
  ❖ cardiac dysrhythmias
  ❖ certain ECG abnormalities, including prolonged QT interval (glossary)
  ❖ hyperthyroidism.

◆ Adreno-ceptor agonists will worsen some conditions:
  ❖ diabetes
  ❖ acute angle glaucoma
  ❖ prostatic hypertrophy
  ❖ hyperthyroidism.

◆ Long-acting beta$_2$ agonists are not advised for patients whose asthma is deteriorating (BNF 2007).

◆ Lower doses may be required if renal function is poor.

- **Pregnant** women should be reassured that poorly controlled asthma is more likely to harm the fetus than inhaled bronchodilators at prescribed doses. Manufacturers advise against use of formoterol.

- **Breastfeeding.** Adrenoceptor agonists probably enter breastmilk. Risks and benefits should be evaluated. Breastfeeding probably helps to protect the infant from asthma and allergy. Avoid formoterol.

- Record prescriptions. Illegal use to enhance absorption of inhaled cocaine has been reported

- **Hypersensitivity responses**, including paradoxical bronchospasm, with any component of the product, preclude further use.

Interactions (summary): Beta blockers should be avoided for patients with bronchospasm (BNF 2007). They prevent adrenoceptor agonists relieving symptoms.

Corticosteroids and theophylline/aminophylline are often co-prescribed with adrenoceptor agonists. However, they increase the risks of: potassium loss and fluid retention.

Cardiac dysrhythmias are more likely with co-administration of: diuretics, digoxin, antipsychotics, theophylline/aminophylline, some antidepressants (particularly MAOIs), some gaseous anaesthetics, and other stimulants, including amphetamines, cocaine, 'cold cures'.

Betel nut may worsen asthma (Fugh-Berman 2000).

Antimuscarinic bronchodilators: Ipratropium may be administered by inhaler or nebuliser as short-term relief for patients with COPD or to manage severe asthma. Inhaled tiotropium may be included in maintenance regimens of patients with COPD (Cooper & Tashkin 2005). Antimuscarinics are described with antiemetics.

9 Corticosteroids

Corticosteroids suppress inflammation, allergy and the immune system. They prevent and relieve the symptoms of many conditions.

Actions: Corticosteroid medications are synthetic versions of the hormones secreted by the adrenal cortex. These hormones are essential for maintenance of several systems, particularly the cardiovascular system. They also play a major role in the body's response to stress and starvation. Their actions are grouped into:

◆ glucocorticoid effects, including metabolic changes and anti-inflammatory actions.

◆ mineralocorticoid effects, mainly retention of salt and water. Most steroids mimic the actions of aldosterone, and increase sodium reabsorption in the kidneys, in exchange for potassium or hydrogen ions.

Indications:

◆ **Symptom control**: asthma, allergic rhinitis, rheumatoid arthritis and related connective tissue disorders, temporal arteritis, inflammatory bowel disease, inflammatory skin conditions, emesis following chemotherapy, chronic pain, anaphylactic shock.

◆ **Prevention**: transplant rejection, respiratory distress in the newborn, cerebral oedema.

◆ **Treatment**: certain cancers, some blood disorders, nephrotic syndrome.

◆ **Replacement therapy** in Addison's disease (under-activity of the adrenal cortex).

Administration: Regular medication reviews are needed to ensure doses are kept to the minimum necessary to manage the underlying condition (NICE 2004a, BTS 2005).

Inhaled beclometasone, budesonide daily doses >800mcg (adult) >400mcg (child) are associated with systemic (general) side effects (Lipworth & Wilson 2002). These side effects are seen at half these doses for fluticasone (BTS 2005). Some 'high dose' regimens include daily doses up to 2mg and 1mg (fluticasone). Clinical improvement should be observed within 3–7 days. As lung function improves, more inhaled drug is absorbed, making adverse effects more likely. The type of inhaler device may alter drug absorption, by as much as 500% (Wilson et al. 1999); these should not be interchanged without authorisation of prescriber (see bronchodilators and Box 8.1).

Oral prednisolone: side effects are more likely if daily dose >7.5mg. Severe disease may necessitate much higher doses. Most, if not all, the daily dose should be administered, with breakfast, before 9.00 a.m. This mimics the body's natural secretion of corticosteroids, and minimises the risk of adrenal suppression (below).

Topical applications: systemic adverse effects are likely when: potent corticosteroids (e.g. beclometasone 0.1%, clobetasol propionate 0.05%) are applied to extensive areas of skin for prolonged periods; skin is inflamed; occlusive dressings are applied, including disposable nappies.

Local adverse drug reactions: CORTICOSTEROIDS

Route	Potential Local Adverse Effects	Suggested Management
Oral	Irritation to lining of upper gastrointestinal tract	Take with milk or food plus full glass of water and remain upright for 30 minutes. (Box 1.1)
Intravenous injection	Injection of dexamthasone administered for chemotherapy-induced emesis or hydrocortisone as sodium phosphate ester is often accompanied by pain and a 'tingling' sensation in the perineal area	Warn patients
Intramuscular injection	Muscle atrophy at the injection site. Local reactions	Use each site only once and document
Inhaler devices (Box 8.1)	Oral candidiasis (thrush) Oral, laryngeal and pharyngeal irritation, mucosal or muscle atrophy may cause cough, hoarseness, speech difficulties Irritation of peri-oral skin Thirst Tongue hypertrophy (rare)	Spacer devices may decrease oral candidiasis, but increase cough (Dubus et al. 2001) Mouth rinsing may reduce candidiasis and systemic absorption Cough can be minimised by pre-treatment with an inhaled beta$_2$ agonist (BNF 2007) Monitor children for speech development Inspect the oral cavity regularly
Intranasal applications	Headache, nausea, urticaria, rebound congestion, perforation of the nasal septum, loss of sense of smell, nose bleeds, due to atrophy of the lining of the nose	Restrict administration to recommended doses, particularly if patients are using beclometasone and budesonide nasal sprays without prescription
Skin	Spread of infection, acne, dermal atrophy, hirsuitism, depigmentation, perioral dermatitis, telangiectases and striae	Avoid application to the face and broken skin without specialist advice. Restrict non-prescription use to adults, maximum of 5–7 days
Intra-articular injections	Osteonecrosis, tendon rupture, and infection	Consult specialist regarding exercises and avoidance of weight bearing
Rectal administration (Box 1.2)	Local pain, burning, rectal bleeding, delayed healing	Avoid if the patient has bowel obstruction, recent gastrointestinal surgery, bleeding tendencies or infection

Ophthalmic application	Infections, thinning or perforation of cornea and sclera, glaucoma and cataracts	Specialist supervision
Ear drops	Sensitivity reactions	Avoid prolonged use

(BNF 2007, Karch 2006, Griffiths & Jordan 2002)

Adverse effects:

Impaired immunity: Corticosteroids act on all aspects of the immune system. They:

◆ decrease inflammatory mediators (including prostaglandins) reducing pain and swelling.

◆ inhibit white cell migration to sites of tissue damage and microbial invasion, increasing the risk of infections.

◆ block macrophage (glossary) activation, increasing the risk of reactivation of dormant infections, particularly tuberculosis.

◆ suppress the immune response, increasing the severity of existing infections and, possibly, the spread of malignancies (Aronson 2006).

◆ shrink lymphoid tissue.

◆ decrease proliferation of fibroblasts (glossary), collagen and new blood vessels, reducing healing and scar tissue formation.

Nutrition and metabolism: Corticosteroids increase the availability of glucose, to protect the brain and heart during starvation. Fats and proteins are broken down to provide this glucose. However, when it is not used as energy, the excess glucose is converted into central adipose deposits.

Protein breakdown and vulnerability to infection can affect any of the body's organs, including bones, skin, the GI tract, muscles.

Fluid and electrolyte imbalance, due to mineralocorticoid actions. Sodium retention promotes fluid retention, which causes oedema, weight gain, hypertension and congestive heart failure (Slordal & Spigset 2006), and can also affect the eyes. Cardiovascular risk profile may be worsened by long-term therapy.

Neurological: Patients with Addison's disease or Cushing's syndrome may show signs of mental illness, which disappear following treatment.

Adrenal suppression/ insufficiency: This potentially life-threatening condition is due to disruption of the hypothalamic/pituitary/adrenal (HPA) axis, which controls the production of steroids. Normally, stress increases secretion of corticosteroids, up to tenfold. However, the adrenals of patients prescribed long-term corticosteroids are unable to respond as normal. This is attributed to the suppression of the adrenal cortex by prescribed corticosteroids; these disrupt the regular feedback system and remove the normal stimulation to the adrenals (Figure 9.1). Eventually, the adrenals atrophy, and are no longer able to increase hormone secretion in response to stress.

Problems arise when individuals with adrenal suppression and insufficiency are exposed to severe stress e.g. infection, trauma, surgery, or abruptly discontinue therapy. Problems can emerge after 1 weeks' therapy and persist for up to a year after discontinuation.

Steroids also inhibit secretion of oestrogens and androgens.

67

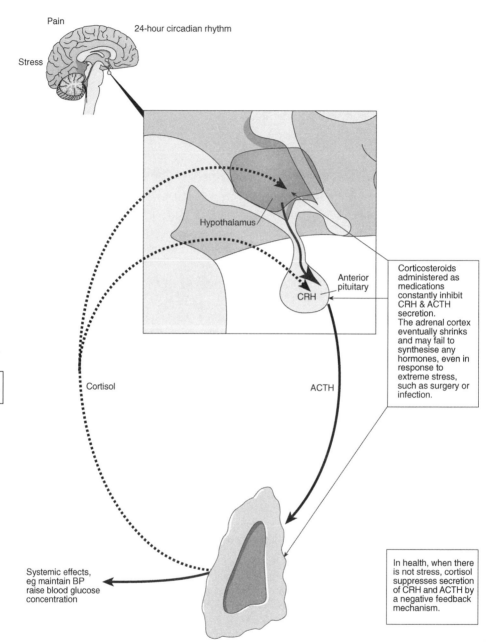

Pain

Stress

24-hour circadian rhythm

Hypothalamus

Anterior pituitary

CRH

Corticosteroids administered as medications constantly inhibit CRH & ACTH secretion. The adrenal cortex eventually shrinks and may fail to synthesise any hormones, even in response to extreme stress, such as surgery or infection.

Cortisol

ACTH

Systemic effects, eg maintain BP raise blood glucose concentration

In health, when there is not stress, cortisol suppresses secretion of CRH and ACTH by a negative feedback mechanism.

Figure 9.1   The hypothalmic/pituitary/adrenal axis

Adverse effects: implications for practice: CORTICOSTEROIDS

Short courses of high doses for emergencies cause fewer adverse effects than prolonged courses using lower doses. If therapy has lasted <1 week, or is confined to a single large dose, problems are not anticipated. Many adverse effects, for example, those related to nutrition, only arise with long-term therapy. Individuals differ in their susceptibility.

Potential Problem	Suggestions for Prevention and Management
Impaired immunity	
Increased risk of infections	Teach good hand washing techniques
	Monitor body temperature at 5–6 p.m. daily
	Contact doctor at first signs of infection, as timely antibiotics may be important
	Take swabs at earliest opportunity
	Avoid exposure to infectious disease
	Contact prescriber on exposure to chickenpox or measles.
Immunisations for patients prescribed oral or rectal corticosteroids	Avoid live vaccines e.g. BCG, MMR, yellow fever and oral typhoid vaccines during treatment and for at least 3 months afterwards. (see DH 2006 for doses)
Replacement regimens, inhaled and topical corticosteroids do not contra-indicate routine immunisations	Inactivated vaccines are likely to be less effective e.g. tetanus, diphtheria, pertussis, hepatitis B (DH 2006)
Reactivation of latent infection e.g. tuberculosis, amoebiasis, *Herpes simplex* and fungal or viral eye infections (see cautions)	Obtain a detailed history of previous infections, particularly in contact lens wearers
	Monitor patients previously exposed to tuberculosis
Nutrition and metabolism	
Increased appetite: as in starvation, or a full day without food, there is a tendency to eat convenience foods	Encourage a well balanced, low calorie diet. Ask dietician to provide diet plan
	Monitor intake by asking patient to record intake for 24-hour periods
	Weigh patient weekly (see antipsychotics)
Hyperglycaemia/diabetes (without ketosis)	Monitor blood glucose concentrations regularly and if thrush appears on the skin
Increased cholesterol and triglyceride concentrations	Monitor lipid profile
Redistribution of body fat, to trunk and face	Measure waist circumference regularly (see antipsychotics). This predicts cardiovascular risk
Altered body image	Consider impact on compliance and risk of abrupt withdrawal (below). Minimise weight gain

Bones	
Osteoporosis & fractures. Most bone loss occurs in the first 6 months of therapy. Doses >7.5mg for >3 months indicate significant risk (BNF 2007) Corticosteroids decrease the activity of the cells which form bone (the osteoblasts), and increase the activity of the cells which breakdown bone (the osteoclasts). They also increase calcium elimination and oppose the actions of vitamin D	Encourage patient to eat foods high in calcium, to ensure intake is 1500mg/day. Vitamin D intake should be 400 IU/day. A pint of milk contains about 600mg calcium, but very little vitamin D. This is obtained from oily fish e.g. salmon, or synthesised during exposure to sunlight Suggest calcium and vitamin D supplementation, on initiation of long-term therapy, together with monitoring for vitamin D intoxication Encourage moderate exercise Consider need for further protective measures Bone densiometry on initiation of therapy (Schimmer & Parker 2006) Be prepared to administer bisphosphonates, calcitrol (a vitamin D analogue), HRT or androgens for prevention or treatment of osteoporosis.
Osteonecrosis (at any age). This may progress to joint destruction. The head of femur is the commonest site	Sudden onset of joint pain and stiffness should be reported immediately
Growth or puberty delay Any delay may be temporary, with 'catch-up' after 1 year	Plot height and weight on centile charts at regular intervals. Remind patients that untreated serious illness reduces final height. Discuss specialist referral if growth is slowed. Discuss morning-only administration, with prescriber. Be prepared to discuss alternate day therapy, and its impact on compliance. Advise that termination of therapy before puberty will probably allow predicted height to be achieved.
Skin (particularly topical preparations)	
Poor wound healing Thinning of the skin, striae, bleeding, bruising	Consult podiatrist regarding foot-care. Anticipate poor healing and contact wound care specialists promptly. Take swabs if healing delayed. Increased vigilance of pressure areas. Evaluate pressure damage risk regularly. Avoid friction and shearing forces on the skin, for example, teach patients in the correct use of moving and handling aids (glide sheets) when moving along the bed/chair. Allow extra time for procedures involving tissue handling, such as transfer to hoist, care of infusion sites. Ensure good communication within the multidisciplinary team: for example, orthopaedic surgeons, plaster technicians or nurses applying plaster casts, need to be aware that the patient is prescribed corticosteroids, and adjust treatment, if possible.

Increase in body hair (hirsuitism) and acne	Provide advice on managing acne
Contact allergy and itching	Withhold therapy until prescriber has been informed.
Gastrointestinal tract	
Bleeding from peptic ulceration	Observe and test stools for blood loss
Muscles	
Muscle weakness and fatigue due, in part, to disruption of carbohydrate metabolism	Routine exercise may help to prevent or decrease muscle weakness Assess activities such as rising from a chair. Inform prescriber if this worsens Monitor respiratory function Review serum potassium concentrations
Cramps	Check eletrolytes if cramps occur
Fluid and electrolyte disorders	
Fluid retention	Limit sodium intake to 2.4g/day Fluid balance records and daily weighing are important during initiation of therapy
Loss of potassium, causing muscle weakness, depression, constipation, cardiac complications	Venous blood samples to monitor electrolytes Encourage foods that are high in potassium e.g. raisins, bananas, meat
Hypertension, some 20% of patients develop hypertension (Sholter & Armstrong 2000)	Foods rich in salt should be avoided, except with replacement regimens. Condiments and processed foods are high in sodium. Avoid sodium-containing medicines and liquorice Monitor blood pressure regularly
Congestive heart failure	Observe for breathlessness (see beta blockers)
Thrombosis Increased numbers of red cells and possibly platelets make thrombosis more likely	Monitor full blood count and cardiovascular risk factors

Eyes (particularly eye drops or if creams applied close to eyes)

Changes in metabolism or fluid retention make the eyes vulnerable to: ◆ **increased intraocular pressure and glaucoma** ◆ **cataracts or clouding of vision (particularly children)** ◆ **infections e.g. *Herpes simplex*, fungal infections**	For all routes of administration, regular eye examinations are needed to detect changes before permanent eye damage occurs. Arrange appointments on initiation of therapy, after 6 months, then at least yearly if dose of prednisolone >10mg/day (Schimmer & Parker 2006)

Neurological

Emotional changes such as moodiness, depression, euphoria, restlessness, insomnia, hallucinations, suicidal ideation (Schimmer & Parker 2006)	Monitor behaviour. Advise parents to be alert for difficulties Discuss the substitution of enteric coated tablets with prescriber (Aronson 2006) Consider the possibility of steroid psychosis and refer as necessary
Memory impairment	Monitor cognitive function Review therapy in patients with dementia
Steroid abuse/ dependence	Refer patients who resist dose reductions

Reproductive system

Changes in menstrual cycle **Impotence**	Advise patients of potential problems. Refer to prescriber

Adrenal suppression

Adrenal insufficiency **Signs and symptoms include:** **weakness, nausea, weight loss, hypoglycaemia, dehydration, electrolyte imbalance and hypotension**	**Prevention** ◆ Administer medication before 9.00 a.m. ◆ Monitor pulse, blood pressure, electrolytes and glucose regularly, particularly when reducing doses or changing preparations. ◆ Re-check if bruises appear. ◆ After 1 week's use, advise against sudden discontinuation of therapy. ◆ For children using high dose therapy, arrange for venous blood samples to be taken regularly for morning plasma cortisol measurements. A low concentration indicates adrenal suppression and need for further monitoring. **Management** ◆ Inform prescriber. Be prepared to increase dose in the immediate term. ◆ Mark notes clearly

Adrenal crisis is characterised by nausea, vomiting, abdominal pain, exhaustion, dehydration, hypotension and shock	**Prevention** ◆ Be prepared to increase dose to meet additional demands, such as infection. ◆ Ensure surgical and anaesthetic teams are informed of any current or past use of corticosteroids. ◆ Advise carrying a 'steroid card' and wearing a medi alert bracelet to inform emergency workers of medication. **Management** ◆ Inform prescriber urgently. Ensure intravenous hydrocortisone is available. ◆ Mark notes clearly
Withdrawal of therapy	
Flare-up of underlying condition	Supervise gradual withdrawal of therapy, particularly if dose of prednisolone above 7.5mg/day. If disease is likely to recur, reduction of prednisolone may be 1mg/month (Aronson 2006)
Fever, malaise, 'aches and pains', anorexia	Supervise transition from oral to inhaled administration and conversion to alternate day therapy
Raised intracranial pressure (rare)	Continue to monitor patients for possible adrenal insufficiency (above) for a year after discontinuation

Rare adverse effects include: vasculitis, cardiac dysrhythmia, benign intracranial hypertension, damage to bowel, pancreatitis, kidney stones.

73

Cautions and contra-indications:

◆ **Presence of infections.** Infections may 'flare up', including HIV/AIDS, previous TB, wound infection, eye infections, *Herpes simplex*.

◆ **Conditions which will be exacerbated**: hypertension, diabetes, heart failure, osteoporosis, glaucoma, epilepsy, mood disorders, pressure sores, diverticulitis.

◆ **Conditions where potassium loss** will prove dangerous: liver failure.

◆ Situations where **muscle weakening** could be problematic: recent myocardial infarction, muscle wasting, elderly, bedridden.

◆ **Masking** of serious symptoms: peptic ulcer, inflammatory bowel disease, pneumonia.

◆ Evaluate long-term use in patients already at high risk of stroke or heart attack.

◆ **Lower** doses are needed in patients unable to eliminate drugs at the normal rate: hypothyroidism, liver failure, renal failure, elderly. Calculation of steroid exposure should include all routes of administration.

◆ **Pregnancy.** The risks of intrauterine growth retardation from repeated courses of intra-muscular corticosteroids, administered to prevent respiratory distress of the new-born, are under investigation. When corticosteroids are administered for severe maternal disease, benefits are likely to outweigh risks. Most prednisolone (unlike dexametasone) is inactivated by the placenta.

◆ **Breastfeeding:** avoid if >40mg prednisolone/day (or equivalent) administered. Doses below those causing systemic side effects are considered safe.

Interactions (summary): Corticosteroids interact with many drugs.
Adverse effects may be intensified:

◆ Increased risk of gastrointestinal bleeding: alcohol, anticoagulants, aspirin, NSAIDs.

◆ Increased fluid retention and hypertension: beta$_2$ agonists, NSAIDs, sodium-containing preparations, oestrogens, liquorice, ginseng, some Asian herbal mixtures.

◆ Increased potassium depletion: beta$_2$ agonists, diuretics, digoxin, laxatives.

The effects of some regimens are **antagonised**: anti-epileptics, anti-diabetics, anti-hypertensives, growth hormone, intra-uterine contraceptive devices.

The bioavailability of corticosteroids is effectively reduced by:

◆ co-administration with antacids, within 2 hours.

◆ carbamazepine, phenytoin, rifampicin, theophylline.

The bioavailability of corticosteroids is effectively increased by:

◆ erythromycin, ketoconazole, itraconazole, ciclosporin, some anti-virals.

Contributor

Howard Griffiths RN, BSc, MSc, PGCE (FE), RNT. Clinical Practice Tutor, School of Health Science, Swansea University

10 Antipsychotics

Antipsychotics are often an important component of medical management for people with serious and enduring mental illness, including schizophrenia (RCP 2003) and mania or bipolar disorder (NICE 2006b). They are also prescribed for short-term management of disturbed behaviour.

Actions: Antipsychotics reduce auditory hallucinations and modify behaviour by blocking the actions of neurotransmitters in the central nervous system.

◆ Traditional antipsychotics, such as haloperidol, chlorpromazine, flupentixol, fluphenazine, trifluoperazine, zuclopenthixol exert their effects mainly via dopamine (D_2) receptors. They carry a high risk of posture and movement disorders.

◆ Clozapine acts differently: it exerts its antipsychotic effects by blocking serotonin ($5HT_2$) receptors. It causes fewer posture and movement problems, but there are other serious adverse effects.

◆ Newer drugs, such as olanzapine, quetiapine, risperidone, sertindole, zotepine act on both types of receptors, and have a wide range of adverse effects.

Antipsychotics, to varying degrees, also act on the receptors of the autonomic nervous system (both sympathetic and parasympathetic), histamine receptors and ion channels (Healy 2004).

Administration: **Oral preparations** should be administered at the same time(s) each day with full glass of water. Avoid administration of antacids, kaolin (possibly orlistat) within 2 hours of oral medication.

Liquid and orodispersible formulations are absorbed more rapidly than tablets, which is useful in urgent situations (Currier & Simpson 2001). Liquid haloperidol cannot be mixed with tea or coffee. If mixed with water, orange juice or black coffee, liquid risperidone must be taken immediately. Olanzapine and risperidone are available as orodispersible tablets (unsuitable for people with phenylketonuria). Olanzapine, but not risperidone, can be taken with drinks containing milk.

Different brands or formulations of the same drug should not be interchanged without consulting prescriber or pharmacist.

Depot preparations are prescribed for clients who fail to respond to oral medication due to non-adherence. Depot injections are administered every 1–4 weeks, into a large muscle mass, such as the lateral thigh, ventrogluteal or dorsogluteal sites (Figures 10.1, 10.2). The deltoid muscle is unsuitable.

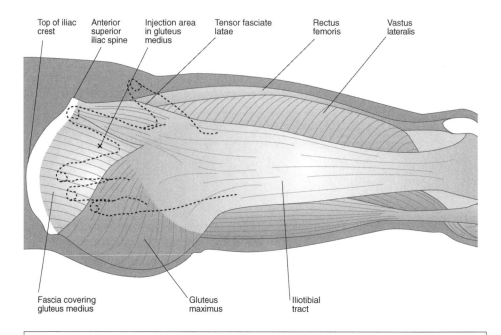

Authorities consider the ventrogluteal site preferable to the dorsogluteal site, because there are fewer nerves and muscles in close proximity (Roger & King 2000, Smith *et al.* 2008). This site is suitable for elderly patients (Hayes *et al.* 2003).

Figure 10.1   The ventrogluteal site: the lateral side of the thigh. Note the two muscles inserted into the iliotibial tract

Sites are rotated and documented. After aspirating, injections (up to 2–3ml) are administered deeply and slowly with a Z-track technique (Figure 10.3).

To avoid erratic absorption, injections should not be administered into fat or fibrous tissue. Depot preparations take weeks to be fully effective and remain in the body for several months.

Store medication below 25°C, away from moisture and light. Discard any which has become discoloured or been frozen. Store long-acting risperidone injection in the refrigerator. Store away from children.

Adverse effects:

♦ **Posture and movement disorders** can occur with all antipsychotics and are inevitable consequences of blocking dopamine receptors in the basal ganglia. These are collections of neurones lying deep within the cerebral hemispheres. They programme and plan movement or convert ideas into voluntary movements. They send impulses to areas of the cerebral cortex linked to the extrapyramidal tracts, which control muscle tone, tension and rigidity. Their neurotransmitters include dopamine, acetylcholine, GABA. Disorders arise when the balance between these is disrupted, whether by drugs or disease (e.g. Parkinson's disease, Huntingdon's chorea, possibly schizophrenia). Amphetamines and cocaine exacerbate any problems.

Injections are placed above an imaginary line joining the 2 bony landmarks (the greater trochanter and the posterior spine of the iliac crest), and above the buttock area

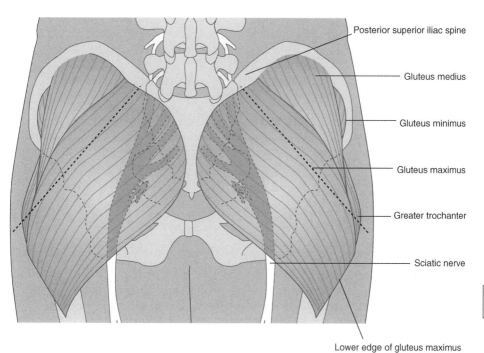

Posterior superior iliac spine

Gluteus medius

Gluteus minimus

Gluteus maximus

Greater trochanter

Sciatic nerve

Lower edge of gluteus maximus

The sciatic nerve usually lies beneath the muscle piriformis.
In some people part of this nerve emerges above (0.5%) or within (12.2%) the muscle. In this unusual position, the nerve is vulnerable to damage from injections placed in the 'upper, outer quadrant' of the buttock.

The dorsogluteal (or buttock) area contains much adipose tissue, which can extend below the gluteal muscles. This can cause confusion when dividing the area into quadrants to locate the dorsogluteal injection site, and allow an injection to be placed too low i.e. close to the sciatic nerve.

Figure 10.2   The dorsugluteal site: the superficial muscles of the gluteal region

◆ **Neurological.** Antipsychotics act on several receptors in the brain, including his-tamine and acetylcholine (muscarinic) receptors, causing sedation and impairing cognition, to a varying extent. Amelioration of psychotic symptoms by dopamine antagonists is often associated with blunting of emotions. Other problems, such as obsessive compulsive disorders, may arise with clozapine therapy. Reduction of activity of the central nervous system may extend to the brain stem and hypo-thalamus, affecting regulatory functions.

◆ **Cardiovascular disturbance.** Antipsychotics may:
  ❖ block anti-muscarinic (parasympathetic) receptors, which increases heart rate

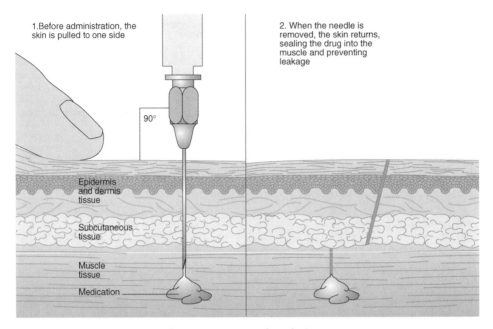

1. Before administration, the skin is pulled to one side

2. When the needle is removed, the skin returns, sealing the drug into the muscle and preventing leakage

90°

Epidermis and dermis tissue

Subcutaneous tissue

Muscle tissue

Medication

Figure 10.3 Z track technique

- ❖ block the sympathetic nervous system, reducing blood pressure (glossary: adrenergic receptors)
- ❖ block the cardiac conduction system, causing heart block (glossary)
- ❖ alter potassium movements in heart muscle, which may make the heart muscle unstable and lead to cardiac dysrhythmias. This may cause a prolonged QT interval (glossary), indicating risk of cardiac events.
- ❖ disrupt the clotting system (clozapine)
- ❖ impact on cardiovascular risk factors: hyperglycaemia, obesity, altered lipid profile, dehydration.

◆ **Nutrition and metabolism.** Drugs acting on serotonin receptors affect appetite and eating behaviour. However, antipsychotics may also alter metabolism, reducing the effectiveness of insulin, raising blood glucose, lipid concentrations and blood pressure. Some clients have developed diabetes without becoming obese.

◆ **Gastrointestinal problems.** Anti-muscarinic actions reduce all secretions and depress gastrointestinal motility.

◆ **Genito-urinary system.** Prolactin secretion is normally held in check by dopamine. Most antipsychotics block the actions of dopamine, thereby facilitating increased prolactin secretion. Prolactin promotes breast growth and impairs fertility. Antipsychotics also disrupt the autonomic nervous system, which controls the genito-urinary system.

(See anti-emetics for anti-muscarinic actions and actions of procyclidine.)

Adverse effects: implications for practice (Jordan *et al.* 2004): Many of the problems below are common to most therapeutic regimens. Problems confined to certain drugs are indicated.

A pre-therapy assessment of all body systems should be undertaken.

Potential Problem	Suggestions for Prevention and Management
Posture and movement disorders	
Acute dystonic reactions, including spasm of muscles in neck, face, jaw, tongue or back, difficulty swallowing or speaking, oculogyric crises or facial grimacing **Usually occur within the first 1–48 hours of use, but sometimes a week later** **Risk increases with dose and emotional disturbance**	Observe tongue movements to detect earliest signs. Remain with patient to reduce fear and observe airway. On diagnosis, anti-muscarinics are administered as quickly as possible (usually intra-muscular procyclidine, into anterolateral thigh, figure 21.1). Relief is usually obtained within 30 minutes. Oral anti-muscarinics are continued. It may be important to identify spurious requests for anti-muscarinics (interactions).
Akathisia may present as subjective feelings of restlessness, inability to keep still, anxiety, insomnia, apprehension, helplessness, agitation, confusion, anger or even violence **Time to onset ranges between hours and months** **Tardive akathisia may be irreversible** **Prevalence: 18–75% (lower with clozapine)**	Seek medication review. Record any abnormal movements, feet shuffling and reports of restlessness. Distinguish from mannerisms, particularly in clients with learning difficulties. Administer and report Barnes' akathisia scale (Barnes 1989). Discuss dosage reduction with prescriber. Procyclidine, propranolol (see beta blockers), benzodiazepines may be prescribed.
Parkinsonism may develop gradually, over several weeks **Clients develop:** ◆ **mask-like facies/ expression** ◆ **bradykinesia, shuffling** ◆ **stooping** ◆ **tremor at rest** ◆ **muscle rigidity**	Distinguish from depression. Observe when walking for: ◆ reduced movements (e.g. arm swings), ◆ small steps, shuffles, feet dragging, bent knees, ◆ stiffness. Administer Simpson Angus scale (Guy 1976, Cunningham Owens 1999). Discuss with prescriber: ◆ dose reduction; ◆ drugs with less effect on dopamine receptors e.g. clozapine ◆ possible referral to speech therapist to assess any swallowing difficulties.

Motor activity, voluntary movements & associated movements are reduced (prevalence 15–35%)	Anti-muscarinics may be prescribed to reduce rigidity (interactions)
Rigidity may affect the right side of the body more than the left	In older people, ensure this is not misdiagnosed as a stroke.
Tremor (may be asymetric) **Problems may be more severe if lithium or valproate co-prescribed**	Observe and monitor finger movements. Place a sheet of paper on outstretched fingers. Report if: ◆ vibration >1 inch ◆ tremor interferes with activities, for example, tying shoelaces, drinking, writing. Discuss the possibility of Parkinsonism.
Tardive dyskinesia starts weeks or years after initiation of therapy and may be irreversible. Clients develop abnormal involuntary movements, constant chewing, grimacing, blinking **Prevalence estimates vary 0.5–65%** **History of ECT increases risk** **Drug withdrawal worsens the condition short term** **Tardive dystonia is an further late-onset syndrome**	Screening: ◆ Ask client to protrude tongue gently for 30 seconds and observe for a fine tremor. ◆ Administer the AIMS scale regularly. ◆ Report earliest signs to prescriber. Prevention: ◆ Avoid dehydration. ◆ Minimise lifetime dose. ◆ Ensure medication is reviewed regularly. Increasing the antipsychotic dose eases tardive dyskinesia temporarily, but worsens the situation long term.
Neuroleptic malignant syndrome. This presents as pyrexia, fluctuating vital signs, sweating, confusion, rigidity (traditional antipsychotics only). This may progress to fluctuating consciousness	Record vital signs. Report immediately. If requested, obtain venous blood sample for measurement of creatinine kinase concentrations, white cell count, liver enzymes and electrolytes.

Neurological	
Sedation, may subside after a few weeks **(Olanzapine, chlorpromazine, pericyazine, clozapine)**	Warn clients in relation to driving, particularly if any alcohol is ingested. Administer medicine before retiring or divide daily dose unequally. Report if sleep is lasting 2 hours more or less than usual. If client is obese and reported to snore heavily, check oxygen saturation and discuss the possibility of sleep apnoea with prescriber.
Insomnia, dreaming (risperidone)	Take medication in the morning.
Poor memory and concentration **Lack of energy**	Report if difficulties or excessive resting are hampering everyday life. Check oxygen saturation in older people.
Cognitive decline, particularly in older patients **Reduced recall**	Monitor mental state Check doses of anti-muscarinics: excessive use impairs cognition.
Depression of respiratory and cardiovascular centres and cough reflex **Hypoxia may cause agitation or even aggression** **Intramuscular administration: risk of respiratory arrest or cardiovascular collapse**	**Continuing care** Assess oxygen saturation in clients with pre-existing respiratory or cardiovascular conditions (interpretation can be unreliable in heavy smokers). If <97%, contact prescriber. Be alert for possible chest infections, especially if client is sedated or hypersalivates. **Rapid tranquilisation** Monitor vital signs, and oxygen saturation, if possible. Client should remain supine for 30 minutes and BP checked before rising (Taylor *et al.* 2005).
Impaired thermoregulation: inability to tolerate cold or hot climates	Maintain environment at a comfortable temperature. Avoid alcohol in hot weather (increases risk of heat stroke).
Risk of seizures (particularly clozapine, zotepine) **Prolonged seizures may follow ECT**	Report seizures. Interactions between antipsychotics and anti-epileptics are complex. Pretreatment EEG may be ordered if there is a history of seizures. Be prepared to co-administer valproate with higher doses of clozapine.
Vision disturbance	
Blurred vision	Advise that blurred vision may subside after 1–2 weeks.
Dry eyes	Assist clients with any artificial tears prescribed.

Difficulties with contact lenses	Advise withholding contact lenses until specialist advice has been sought.
Glaucoma, cataracts, damage to lens and cornea, retinal pigmentation (chlorpromazine, thioridazine)	Ensure clients attend opticians' appointments regularly, to prevent serious eye disease. If night vision is reduced, seek urgent appointment. Minimise sunlight exposure. Use effective dark glasses.

Cardiovascular disturbance

Tachycardia (25% prescribed clozapine) Tachycardia may lead to heart failure or a cardiac event (Box 6.1)	Monitor pulse regularly. Arrange ECG if irregular, >90bpm or <55bpm. Coupled beats or persistent tachycardia in 1st 2 weeks of clozapine therapy indicate need for urgent ECG and medication review. Inquire regarding chest pain or increasing breathlessness.
Cardiac dysrhythmia ECG changes indicate that serious cardiac events may arise suddenly, without further warning signs: ◆ Prolonged QT interval indicates risk of ventricular fibrillation ◆ Heart block may cause bradycardia and 'faints'	Arrange ECGs in accordance with guidelines and individual risks. Pre-breakfast ECGs may be ordered to avoid circadian variations in the T wave. Check risk factors: lithium, carbamazepine and tricyclic therapy, quinine, excitement, stress, heart failure, slow pulse, hypokalaemia, hypomagnesaemia, hypocalcaemia, eating disorders, inherited metabolic abnormalities. Check electrolytes regularly.
Postural hypotension, dizziness, falls Hip fracture risk three times above general population (French et al. 2005)	Monitor BP lying and standing. Report if systolic BP falls by >10% or 20mmHg on standing. (see diuretics) If heart rate also rises by >10%, this indicates dehydration. Advise clients to mobilise slowly.
Heart damage and blood clots (particularly clozapine, affects 0.015–0.188% clients)	Pre-therapy physical examination. Close observation for first few months.
Raised plasma lipids (quetiapine, clozapine, olanzapine, risperidone)	Assess cardiovascular risk factors and lipids (Picchioni & Murray 2007), pre-therapy, at 1 and 6 months, yearly.
Reduced platelet concentration (clozapine, risperidone)	Ask client to report any abnormal bleeding or bruising. For clients using clozapine, full blood counts can be arranged alongside white cell counts.

Nutrition and metabolism	
Weight change: under- or over-eating **Highest risk of weight gain in first 3–20 weeks** **29% using olanzapine, 10% ziprasidone gain >7% body weight after 10 weeks**	Monitor weight, weekly initially. Weigh clients regularly at same time, on same scales, wearing same clothes, after voiding. Report change of 0.5–1kg in 1 week or 2.4kg in 1 month. Measure waist circumference to assess central obesity and cardiovascular risk: should be <88cms (35 inches) in women, <102cm (40 inches) in men. Suggest 'sugar-free' drinks. Check blood glucose and, if indicated, thyroid function if client gains weight. Check blood pressure.
Type 2 diabetes (ketoacidosis rarely) particularly risperidone and olanzapine (Carlson et al. 2006) (see insulin)	Regular measurement of blood glucose within 1 month of starting olanzapine and 3 months for other drugs (NICE 2006c)
Gastrointestinal problems	
Dry mouth causing: ◆ halitosis. ◆ excessive drinking or sucking sweets. ◆ dentures become ill-fitting. ◆ mouth ulcers	Observe inside of mouth for dryness or ulceration. Suggest: ◆ regular sips of water or ice chips (refrigerated tap water is suitable) ◆ sugarless gum, artificial saliva pastilles or spray ◆ avoiding too many sweets ◆ mouthwashes (chlorhexidine reduces plaque formation).
Dental problems due to dry mouth or bruxism (repetitive teeth grinding)	Arrange regular visits to dentist/oral hygienist.
Indigestion or heartburn	Taking oral medication with milk or semisoft food may help.
Constipation: ◆ **Risk of gastrointestinal obstruction.** ◆ **Dopamine antagonists are anti-emetic, which may delay detection.**	Recommend 5 portions (15 ounces/375g) of fruit or vegetables daily. Fruit purees may be helpful (see laxatives). Maintain fluid intake 1–1.5 litres/day, plus normal diet. Encourage activity, if possible. Monitor bowel movements. If bowels open <twice/week, discuss short-term administration of laxatives.
Clozapine increases secretions	
Hypersalivation **Nasal congestion** **Cough** **Secretions may enter the respiratory tract and cause infections**	Suggest sleeping on towels. Avoid anti-muscarinic medication such as procyclidine, hyoscine, if possible. Ensure client has tissues available. Be alert for chest infections.

Nausea (risperidone, clozapine)	Effects may subside after a few weeks. Avoid dopamine antagonist anti-emetics, such as metoclopramide.
Genito-urinary system	
Urine retention, difficulty with urination	Record: incontinence, urgency, pain, burning, bleeding. Undertake urinalysis to detect any infection. If urine stream poor or hesitant, consider enlarged prostate.
Nocturnal enuresis (clozapine)	Suggest morning dosing and reducing fluids before bedtime. Desmopressin may be prescribed.
Reproductive health: breast discomfort; menstrual irregularities; dry vagina; change in libido; erectile/ejaculatory dysfunction; priapism	Discuss with same gender nurse and seek specialist advice. Note duration of amenorrhoea. If over 1 year, discuss bone mineral density measurements with prescriber (Haddad & Wieck 2004). Prolactin concentrations may be measured from venous blood samples.
Fertility may be restored by withdrawal of traditional antipsychotic	Ensure appropriate contraceptive advice is received.
Hypothyroidism (particularly quetiapine)	If client gains weight, becomes cold intolerant or lethargic, consider thyroid function tests.
Injection site	
Pain or fibrous nodules Abscesses may form if large volumes are injected	Discuss oral medication or alternative injection sites with prescriber (Figures 10.1, 10.2). Consider if needles are long enough to penetrate subcutaneous fat (Roger & King 2000) (Figure 10.4). Injections may be less painful if administered slowly (1ml in 10 seconds) *via* small gauge needles and with muscles relaxed e.g. client lying down with toes inverted for dorsogluteal administration. Use filter needles, where possible (Preston & Hegadoren 2004).
Hypersensitivity responses: Most antipsychotics have been implicated in rare cases (chapter 21)	
Blood dyscrasias, including agranulocytosis (0.8% clozapine users, (Picchioni & Murray 2007)) Highest risk 4–10 weeks after initiation	Sore throat, fever and weakness should be reported. Arrange urgent full blood count. Ensure clients prescribed clozapine have venous blood samples collected as arranged by manufacturers. Risks increased with co-administration of carbamazepine, carbimazole or other drugs affecting the bone marrow.

Liver disorders	Liver function tests pre-therapy and during first year of therapy (Taylor et al. 2005).
Contact dermatitis from handling phenothiazines	Immediately wash any skin that contacts phenothiazines
Photosensitivity: sunburn in bright sunlight, even through glass and at cool temperatures (mainly chlorpromazine, thioridazine)	Advise minimising exposure to direct sunlight and covering skin as much as possible e.g. long-sleeved T-shirts, hats. Sunscreen with a high factor (15+) and high stars (at least 4) should be available throughout the year for all skin types.
Therapeutic failure	
Deterioration in mood, restlessness, confusion, irritability or aggression	Discuss expressions of hostility, 'hopelessness', 'helplessness' or 'agitation' with prescriber. Consider akathisia, hypoxia, pain. Measurement of plasma concentration may be possible, particularly clozapine.
'Negative' symptoms and low mood	Discuss expectations of efficacy and adherence (Awad 1999)
Consider patient non-concordance. Fear of adverse events reduces compliance	Monitor and minimise adverse effects as much as possible using a structured profile, available in Jordan et al. (2004), Kane (1999).
Withdrawal reactions	
Abrupt withdrawal can cause vomiting, anorexia, dizziness, insomnia, nightmares, tremors, sweating, nasal congestion, abdominal pain, headache, muscle aches, numbness, psychosis or movement disorders Physical symptoms may begin within 2 days of last dose	Reduce dose gradually over weeks or months. Reduce depot doses in 3 monthly intervals. Advise clients not to discontinue medication abruptly.
Relapse following withdrawal (Whitaker 2004)	Monitor during withdrawal and, for relapse of mental illness, for 2 years afterwards (RCP 2003).

85

Other potential problems include: systemic lupus erythematosis, bone demineralisation, syndrome inappropriate ADH (see anti-depressants)

Cautions and contra-indications:

◆ CNS depression, coma, phaeochromocytoma (glossary).

◆ Reduced white cell count or history of blood dyscrasias.

◆ Clients with liver or kidney impairment require reduced doses.

◆ Antipsychotics exacerbate or complicate management of: diabetes, epilepsy, Parkinsonism, alcoholism, cardiovascular/cerebrovascular disease, respiratory disease, glaucoma, prostatism, thyroid disorders, myasthenia gravis. Tardive dyskinesia may complicate respiratory disease.

◆ **Masking of emesis** is dangerous when GI obstruction (possibly due to faecal impaction caused by anti-muscarinic actions) or lithium toxicity or raised intra-cranial pressure is suspected.

◆ **Pregnancy.** Seek specialist advice prior to conception. When taken in the last trimester, antipsychotics may affect delivery and the neonate: muscle disorders and jaundice may persist. Some authorities advise against breastfeeding (Hardy & Jordan 2002).

◆ **Children.** High risk of posture and movement disorders and weight gain. Avoid during acute febrile illness. Consult manufacturers' literature.

◆ **Older people** (and clients with AIDS) are vulnerable to posture and movement disorders, confusion, cognitive decline and intolerance of hot or cold conditions. Minimal doses may be prescribed. Adult doses are rarely appropriate.

86

Drug interactions (summary): Many prescribed medicines, particularly tricyclic antidepressants, intensify any adverse effects. Close monitoring is needed if SSRIs or lithium are co-prescribed.

Anti-muscarinics may be prescribed to reduce Parkinsonism, but may increase constipation, urine retention, glaucoma, tardive dyskinesia, heat stroke. They may worsen hallucinations or psychosis or cause acute confusional states, known as 'atropine psychosis'. Clients sometimes request repeat administration. Review use, particularly if 'as needed', every 3 months (see anti-emetics for adverse effects). Clozapine manufacturer advises to avoid. Betel nut may counteract the effects of antimuscarinics, causing rigidity or jaw tremor (Fugh-Berman 2000).

Advise against **self-medication**, particularly with 'cold cures', indigestion medicines, antihistamines, amphetamines, St. John's Wort and regular paracetamol. Alcohol increases sedation, hypotension, posture and movement problems. Adverse effects may emerge if clients cease smoking tobacco (possibly cannabis). Clients prescribed clozapine should keep coffee intake fairly constant.

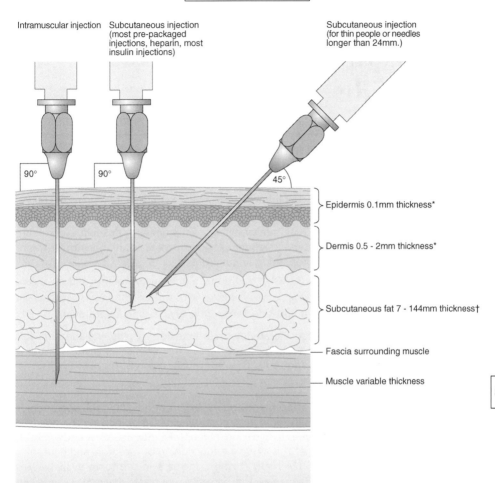

Intramuscular injection

Subcutaneous injection (most pre-packaged injections, heparin, most insulin injections)

Subcutaneous injection (for thin people or needles longer than 24mm.)

90° 90° 45°

Epidermis 0.1mm thickness*

Dermis 0.5 - 2mm thickness*

Subcutaneous fat 7 - 144mm thickness†

Fascia surrounding muscle

Muscle variable thickness

87

*figures for most of the body, in adults. The skin is thicker over the heel and palms.

† Depth of subcutaneous fat depends on the site, the individual, their age, fat stores and gender.

Subcutaneous injections. Subcutaneous fat may be as thin as 7mm. Injections administered at 90 degrees with standard 12.5mm needles could be placed in muscle, affecting absorption and causing tissue atrophy. This problem is most likely to occur in thin adolescent boys with type I diabetes (Shin & Kim 2006). *The depth of the subcutaneous layer should be assessed for each patient. If less than 1 inch (2.4 centimetres) of tissue can be grasped, the subcutaneous injection should be administered at 45 degrees (Berman et al 2008).*

Intramuscular injections. In the dorsogluteal area, depth of subcutaneous fat varies 0.5-6.0 inches (12-144mms.). Depth is more uniform in the ventrogluteal area, usually 37.5mm. (1.6 inches) (Workman 1999). The thick layer of adipose tissue in the dorsogluteal site may cause standard 35mm needles to deposit medication in fat, not muscle, even in women weighing around 8-9 stone (50-60kg) (Cockshott et al 1982). There are fewer problems with the ventrogluteal site (Nisbet 2006). Intramuscular injections are not usually advised in children, but see WHO (2005). The lateral thigh is usually considered the safest site for intramuscular injections.

Absorption from intramuscular or subcutaneous injections may be unusual in both obese and emaciated patients (Wilkinson 2001).

Figure 10.4 Siting of intramuscular and subcutaneous injections

Contributor

Dave Pointon MA, RMN, RNT. Head of Centre for Mental Health Studies (retired), School of Health Sciences, Swansea University

11 Antidepressants: focus on SSRIs

Antidepressants are prescribed to elevate mood. They can be grouped:

◆ Selective serotonin re-uptake inhibitors (**SSRIs**): fluoxetine, paroxetine, sertraline, fluvoxamine, citalopram, escitalopram, duloxetine.

◆ Tricyclic antidepressants (**TCAs**): amitriptyline, imipramine, doxepin, dosulepin (dothiepin) and tricyclic-related: trazodone. Amitriptyline and nortriptyline are prescribed in low doses for neuropathic pain (unlicensed).

◆ Monoamine oxidase inhibitors (MAOIs): traditional e.g. tranylcypromine and reversible e.g. moclobemide.

◆ Others, including mirtazapine, duloxetine, reboxetine, venlafaxine, tryptophan.

Compared to TCAs, SSRIs are better tolerated (less cardiotoxic, less sedative) and safer following overdose (NICE 2004b), but may be less effective for seriously ill clients (Barbui & Hotopf 2001). MAOIs, tryptophan and venlafaxine are usually reserved for specialist use.

Actions: Antidepressants may affect mood and behaviour by adjusting the operation of key neurotransmitters (glossary): serotonin and noradrenaline. SSRIs increase the quantity of serotonin available in key synapses by blocking its reuptake into neurones and removal. TCAs act similarly on noradrenaline. This alters the functioning of receptors and neurones, and tends to normalise circadian (24 hour) rhythms. Increase in serotonin availability is thought to be responsible for mood elevation, anxiety, anorexia, analgesia, change in libido. However, excess may disturb CNS functioning; rarely, extreme excess can produce fever and the 'serotonin syndrome' (below).

Indications: Antidepressants may be an important component of therapy for people with moderate or severe depression (NICE 2004b). Some antidepressants are also prescribed for other conditions, including obsessive compulsive disorders (OCD), bulimia nervosa, impulse disorders. Duloxetine is also prescribed for stress incontinence and diabetic neuropathy, usually under specialist supervision.

Administration: A routine for administration is advisable, for example, paroxetine is best taken once daily, in the morning, with food. Fluoxetine and its main metabolite have unusually long half-lives of up to 10 days (glossary). Therefore, effects may be delayed and fluoxetine will remain in the body several weeks after discontinuation.

Most SSRIs are available as tablets or capsules and liquids. Citalopram oral drops can be mixed with water or orange juice. Different brands and formulations may not be bioequivalent.

Adverse effects:

◆ **Neurological.** Increase in available serotonin or noradrenaline, either alone or by antagonising dopamine, may:
  ❖ over-elevate mood
  ❖ alter behaviour
  ❖ affect posture and movement
  ❖ interfere with melatonin release, disturbing sleep patterns
  ❖ affect ion movements and neurone functioning.

◆ **Other systems.** Serotonin acts on most body systems:
  ❖ Gastrointestinal motility is increased, causing diarrhoea.
  ❖ Arterioles are dilated, reducing peripheral resistance and blood pressure.
  ❖ Platelet activity is decreased, promoting bleeding. SSRIs reduce serotonin entry into platelets; without serotonin, platelets cannot form clots.
  ❖ Antidepressants, to varying degrees, affect other receptors and neurotransmitters, including the autonomic nervous system and dopamine. The skin and the genito-urinary system may be affected.

◆ **Syndrome inappropriate ADH (SIADH).** ADH (anti-diuretic hormone) is secreted from the posterior pituitary in response to water or fluid volume depletion. ADH acts on the collecting ducts of the nephron (Figure 3.1) to conserve water. The overall effect of ADH is to move water from urine into the circulation. Water may then pass into tissue fluid and cells. As a result, a low volume of concentrated urine is produced, while body fluids expand and become more dilute and hyponatraemic (glossary). Occasionally, ADH is secreted in excess in response to surgery or certain drugs (e.g. antidepressants, antipsychotics, some anti-cancer drugs). The resulting water retention allows water to pass into cells, including those in the brain, causing confusion, nausea and even convulsions or coma.

◆ **The serotonin syndrome.** This is a disturbance of the monoamine neurotransmitters of the CNS, probably caused by raised concentrations of serotonin in both the CNS and peripheral tissues. Recognition may not be easy (below).

Adverse effects: implications for practice: SSRIs

More than 80% of people prescribed SSRIs in the community experienced at least one 'bothersome' adverse drug reaction (Hu *et al.* 2004). Less than 1% of inpatients experienced a serious adverse reaction, mainly psychotic and neurological disturbances (Degner *et al.* 2004). Some 10% of the population may be genetically vulnerable to adverse effects, at normal doses.

Potential Problem	Suggestions for Prevention and Management
Neurological problems	
Hypomania/euphoria **Agitation, anxiety, nervousness, amnesia, increased libido/ promiscuity** **Particular care on initiation or increase of therapy or for clients with a history of bipolar disorder**	Distinguish between side effects and 'normal' anxieties, behaviours and sleep loss. Consider alternative causes of overactivity: excess caffeine; non-prescribed stimulants e.g. cold cures; recreational drugs, including cannabis, amphetamines. Provide advice regarding driving, particularly on initiation of therapy, in accordance with BNF. See clients within days of initiation of therapy. Refer any problems to prescriber promptly.
Insomnia	Administer medication earlier in the day. Seek medication review: a more sedating antidepressant may be prescribable.
Panic attacks. Panic symptoms may increase on initiation of therapy	Discuss gradual dose incrementation with prescriber.
Restlessness/akathisia **Subjective feelings of restlessness, inability to keep still, apprehension, helplessness, confusion, anger, aggression or violence, suicidal ideation and self-harm** **Hallucinations, abnormal dreams** **Time to onset ranges between hours and months**	Monitor closely for ideation of violent behaviour or self-harm, particularly during first month of therapy and dose changes. Ask clients to report these feelings (NICE 2004b). Refer to prescriber any clients who appear fidgety, are unable to sit still or complain of inner restlessness. Dose reduction may be needed. Hallucination may indicate that dose is excessive (Aronson 2006). Community prescribers may issue only 1 weeks' medication at any one time.
Tremor affects about 20% clients **Onset usually 1–2 months after initiation**	Observe outstretched hands for tremor before and during therapy. Evaluate impact of tremor on motor activities, such as writing. Discuss intake of: caffeine, amphetamines, bronchodilators. Review drug interactions for possible serotonin syndrome.
Posture and movement disturbances (<1% clients, particularly paroxetine)	Observe for motor signs of restlessness. Acute dystonic reactions are possible (see antipsychotics). Careful monitoring if client is already taking antipsychotics, lithium or valproate.
Sedation (particularly trazodone, TCAs, mirtazapine)	Advise that problems may subside within 7–14 days. Discuss, with prescriber, administration of medication as single dose at evening meal or bedtime.

Somnolence (17% clients prescribed citalopram)	Seek medication review: less sedating antidepressants may be prescribable.
Weakness or apathy, particularly older clients	Refer to prescriber. Dose reduction or change of medication may be necessary.
Headache within 1–2 hours of taking medication	Discuss with prescriber: dividing the dose; administration at bedtime; administration of paracetamol.
Headache, migraine, tinnitus, paraesthesia	Inform prescriber. Seek medication review.
Dizziness, ataxia, vertigo	Consider risk of injury. Check postural hypotension (below).
Fever	Monitor vital signs pre-therapy and regularly. Report, see serotonin syndrome, below.
Yawning, coughing (particularly citalopram)	Advise clients that these are common adverse effects.
Increased risk of seizures, particularly clients suffering from epilepsy	Ensure any anti-epileptic medication is reviewed pre-therapy and regularly. Report any seizures immediately. Obtain venous blood sample to check serum sodium (below).
Vision changes **Blurred vision TCAs, SSRIs** **Glaucoma (more likely with TCAs, but possible with SSRIs)**	Arrange regular appointments with opticians to pre-empt serious eye disease.
Gastrointestinal disturbances	
Nausea (20% of clients), abdominal cramps, Indigestion Serotonin increases the motility of the gut	Administer with food or at bedtime. Discuss with prescriber: dividing the dose; co-administration with antacids. No evidence of any interactions (Baxter 2006). Warn clients of this common problem, and discuss compliance. Problems may subside after a few weeks.
Diarrhoea (fluoxetine, sertraline)	If faecal incontinence or sleep disturbance occur, seek alternative antidepressant.
Constipation (paroxetine, fluvoxamine)	Advise monitoring bowel movements. (See antipsychotics.)
Dry mouth/xerostomia (18% taking citalopram, TCAs)	Advise regular dental inspections. Suggest regular water rinses. (See antipsychotics.)
Taste disturbance (more severe with TCAs)	Warn clients of this potential problem. Advise on mouth care and xerostomia. Advise clients to monitor food intake if this problem develops.

Hypersalivation **Nasal congestion, rhinitis (citalopram)**	If troublesome, seek medication review.
Weight changes ◆ **Anorexia and weight loss (most SSRIs)** ◆ **Weight gain (paroxetine, citalopram, mirtazapine, TCAs)**	Record weight weekly. Monitor intake if changes >0.5–1kg in 1 week or >2.4kg in 1 month. Discuss dietician referral or medication review, with prescriber.
Abnormal glucose concentrations	Ensure clients with diabetes are monitored for hypoglycaemia. Anti-diabetic medication may need review.
Cardiovascular disturbance	
Postural hypotension **Hip fracture risk doubles (French _et al._ 2005)**	Advise standing slowly on initiation of therapy. Check BP lying and standing (see diuretics).
Hypertension (venlafaxine)	Monitor BP pre-therapy and regularly.
Palpitations (6% clients), changes in heart rate **Cardiac dysrhythmias or heart block (glossary) with TCAs** **Possible QT interval prolongation (glossary), with SSRIs particularly citalopram, venlafaxine, TCAs**	Monitor pulse pre-therapy and regularly. Particular care in older adults. Arrange ECG if abnormalities detected or palpitations occur, and following overdose.
Clotting abnormalities	
Bleeding and bruising **Platelet dysfunction** **Vaginal bleeding** **GI bleeds, stroke (particularly the elderly) (van Walraven _et al._ 2001)**	Warn clients to inform prescriber immediately if bleeding occurs or bruises appear. Obtain venous blood sample for full blood count and prothrombin time. Advise against use of NSAIDs, analgesic doses of aspirin.
Skin: Autonomic and immunological disturbance	
Increased sweating	Extra vigilance for pressure areas.
Acne, herpes simplex reactivation	Advise clients to seek treatment at earliest opportunity.

Hair loss (particularly fluoxetine) **Usually transient, and always reversible**	Discuss with prescriber: thyroid function tests; alternative anti-depressants.

Genito-urinary system	
Loss of libido. Increase also possible **Sexual dysfunction (17% of clients), impotence (particularly paroxetine)** **Paroxetine and sertraline delay ejaculation**	Consider impact on adherence to medication regimen and quality of life. Seek advice from prescriber or nurse specialist.
Menstrual irregularities	Advise menstruation may be delayed. Advise clients to maintain records.
Gynaecomastia, galactorrhoea	If troublesome, discuss alternative therapies with prescriber.
Increased frequency of micturition, polyuria	Approach issues tactfully with older clients. Discuss any continence issues arising.
Urine retention	Inquire regarding symptoms of prostatic hypertrophy. Check urine sample for possible infection.

Syndrome inappropriate ADH (SIADH)	
Hyponatraemia (glossary) *May cause:* **Confusion, lethargy, drowsiness, possibly with headache, nausea and fluid retention. This may be due to SIADH** **Problems take 3–120 days to emerge**	Obtain venous blood sample to monitor sodium concentration, particularly older clients taking diuretics in warm weather. Refer urgently if serum sodium <135 mmol/l.

Serotonin syndrome	
Rare but serious. May cause: confusion, agitation, hypomania, euphoria, sweating and shivering, hallucinations, tremor, BP changes, myoclonus (muscle contractions/ shaking (glossary)), diarrhoea, incoordination, eventually progressing to fever and convulsions	Check vital signs and refer to prescriber immediately. Withhold medication. If the serotonin syndrome is not recognised, and the drugs stopped, the condition will deteriorate. *Prevention:* avoid: amphetamines, cocaine, cold cures, alcohol binges, certain prescribed medicines (interactions).

Not all these are present simultaneously	
Hypersensitivity and organ damage (rare) (chapter 21)	
Rash (often itching), which may indicate serious adverse reactions or vasculitis	Warn clients to inform doctor and withhold SSRIs or venlafaxine if a rash appears.
Photosensitivity and sunburn (also with St John's Wort)	Advise covering skin with clothing and high factor, high star sunscreen during exposure to direct sunlight.
Lung damage (rare) **Asthma may be worsened by TCAs**	Inform prescriber if client becomes short of breath. Record medication on client's asthma records.
Withdrawal reaction	
Gastrointestinal upset, headache, flu-like symptoms, panic/anxiety, insomnia, hypomania, agitation, restlessness, confusion, dizziness, sensory disturbance, numbness, fatigue, tremor, depression (Perahia *et al.* 2005) **These symptoms may be confused with the original problems**	Discontinue medication gradually over several weeks or months (minimum 4 weeks), if possible. If symptoms occur, reduce the dose decrements. This is easier with liquid preparations. Obtain detailed history of compliance. Withdrawal reactions may occur following missed doses if drugs with short half-lives are prescribed e.g paroxetine. Advise clients not to miss or delay doses. Fewer problems with fluoxetine, due to its very long half-life.
Therapeutic failure	Some response should be evident within 1 month (longer with fluoxetine). Explore whether dose is too low or client is abandoning treatment without waiting 6–8 weeks. Older people may take longer to respond.

Rare adverse effects include: joint and muscle pains, bone marrow suppression, liver or pancreas damage, angioedema, anaphylaxis, neuroleptic malignant syndrome (see antipsychotics).

Cautions and contra-indications:

◆ Mania, agitation, need for sedation

◆ History of mania

◆ Suicidal ideation

◆ Previous panic attacks may be worsened. Gradual introduction of SSRIs, preferably under specialist supervision, may be possible.

◆ Epilepsy. Close monitoring is essential.

◆ Parkinsonism may be worsened.

- Heart disease and conduction disturbance likely to be worsened (particularly TCAs, venlafaxine).
- Hypertension. Venlafaxine is not used for patients with hypertension or heart disease.
- Bleeding disorders, previous GI bleeds
- Angle-closure glaucoma
- Diabetes. Insulin requirements may change.
- Renal or hepatic impairment or advanced age necessitate lower or less frequent doses. In severe disease, prescribing may be restricted.
- Previous hypersensitivity responses.
- **Pregnancy.** Manufacturers advise prescription only after careful assessment of risks and benefits. Women with established history of mood disorder should be managed by specialists (O'Keane & March 2007). Escitalopram demonstrated toxicity in animal studies. There are reports of possible links with neonatal lung damage (Chambers *et al.* 2006) and, for paroxetine, heart damage (Berard *et al.* 2007). Neonates may experience withdrawal reactions following use in late pregnancy. These include jitteriness, hypoglycaemia, hypothermia and respiratory distress (Aronson 2006).
- **Breastfeeding.** Most manufacturers advise avoid. There is little evidence of harm to healthy term neonates (Hendrick *et al.* 2001). Close observation of the baby's behaviour is essential. Fluoxetine has a greater potential to accumulate, and may be best avoided.
- **People <18.** Fluoxetine may be prescribed with careful monitoring. Most other SSRIs, mirtazepine and venlafaxine are not recommended for depression (CSM warning in BNF 2007).
- **Overdose.** Deaths from SSRI overdose have usually been associated with alcohol or other drugs. Ensure antidepressants, particularly TCAs and MAOIs, are stored securely away from children.

95

Interactions (summary): SSRIs interact with many other medicines. Clients should inform pharmacists of their medication and seek advice before using non-prescription remedies, particularly 'cold cures', 'stimulants', cimetidine and St John's Wort. Alcohol may intensify any sedation. Experts advise limiting intake to one drink/day (Doran 2003). Co-administration of recreational drugs may be dangerous: mania has been reported with co-administration of cannabis or amphetamines, and convulsions with LSD.

Specialists may, occasionally, consider combination of antidepressants. Interactions between SSRIs or TCAs and MAOIs are particularly dangerous.

Co-administration of SSRIs with MAOIs, levodopa, selegiline, St John's Wort, buspirone, sibutramine (for obesity), tramadol, tri-iodothyronine, triptans (for migraine), tryptophan, lithium, cocaine, amphetamines (such as methylphenidate or dexamfetamine prescribed for adult attention deficit disorder) or some antiviral drugs and possibly erythromycin and ECT may induce the serotonin syndrome. Reactions may occur several weeks after withdrawal of fluoxetine.

In those who are genetically susceptible, SSRIs may cause accumulation and toxicity of: antipsychotics, carbamazepine, diazepam, lithium, phenytoin, procyclidine, TCAs, tramadol, warfarin, ropivacaine, some anti-arrhythmics, some antimalarials.

Bleeding, without change in prothrombin time, is more likely if NSAIDs, clozapine, phenothiazines or anticoagulants are co-administered.

Manufacturers advise caution if **ECT** is co-administered. Seizures may be prolonged with fluoxetine. Antidepressants and anaesthetic agents may interact, particularly in older people and those with heart disease. TCAs and MAOIs increase the risk of cardiovascular complications. Ensure anaesthetist is informed of drugs and doses.

Tricyclics (TCAs) share many of the adverse reactions of antipsychotics, e.g. urine retention, constipation, vision disturbance. When compared to SSRIs, they cause more sedation, weight gain, constipation, cardiac dysrhythmia, and are more likely to worsen diabetes or asthma. Their cardiotoxicity makes them dangerous in overdose and unsuitable for people who have recently suffered mycardial infarctions, have cardiac arrhythmia, liver disease or mania.

St John's Wort is an unlicensed herbal remedy for depression. It interacts with many prescribed drugs, including SSRIs. It causes photosensitivity.

Contributor

Mo Afzal BSc (Hons), RMN, MSc (Econ), PGCE (FE). MBA Learning and Development Manager, Substance Misuse Services, Birmingham and Solihull Mental Health Trust

12 Anti-emetics

Emesis (nausea and vomiting) causes serious physiological disturbances and emotional distress. Once the cause has been established, emesis should be alleviated as soon as possible, using a holistic approach, including prescribed anti-emetics.

When caring for patients with emesis, the full range of causes and contributory factors should be considered, including drugs: opioids, chemotherapy, stimulants (adrenaline, cold cures, beta$_2$ agonists, theophylline), iron tablets, digoxin, NSAIDs, SSRIs, antibiotics, valproate, anti-Parkinson agents, anaesthetics, anti-muscarinics, thyroid hormones; herbal remedies, such as black cohosh, garlic, *Ginkgo biloba*, milk thistle, valerian; recreational drugs, such as alcohol, amphetamines, cocaine, LSD (Figure 12.1).

The vomiting reflex involves many nerves and neurotransmitters, which accounts for the wide variety of drugs used to manage emesis.

Actions: Several very different drugs block the neurotransmitters controlling the areas of the brain and gut responsible for emesis (Figure 12.1). Anti-emetics can be grouped:

◆ **Antihistamines**, for example cyclizine, cinnarizine, promethazine, levomepromazine, and **anti-muscarinics,** for example hyoscine. Procyclidine, orphenadrine are antiuscarinics, mainly prescribed for drug-induced Parkinsonism. These drugs act on both histamine and muscarinic receptors.

◆ **Dopamine antagonists**, for example metoclopramide, domperidone, haloperidol, trifluoperazine, prochlorperazine and other phenothiazines. Some of these are also prescribed as antipsychotics, usually at lower doses.

◆ **5HT$_3$-antagonists,** (serotonin antagonists) for example ondansetron, granisetron, dolasetron, tropisetron, block the excess serotonin released by disturbance of bowel, platelets or brain stem, particularly following radiotherapy of the GI tract.

◆ Corticosteroids, for example dexametasone, are also appetite stimulants.

◆ Cannabinoids, for example nabilone, can help prevent emesis associated with chemotherapy and AIDS.

Aprepitant, octreotide are prescribed in specific circumstances.

Indications: Choice of anti-emetic depends on the cause of emesis (Table 12.1). Anti-emetics are more likely to be needed for younger women, long-term users of alcohol, gynaecological surgery, those with histories of emesis, migraine, anxiety, fatigue or travel sickness (Bartlett & Koczwara 2002).

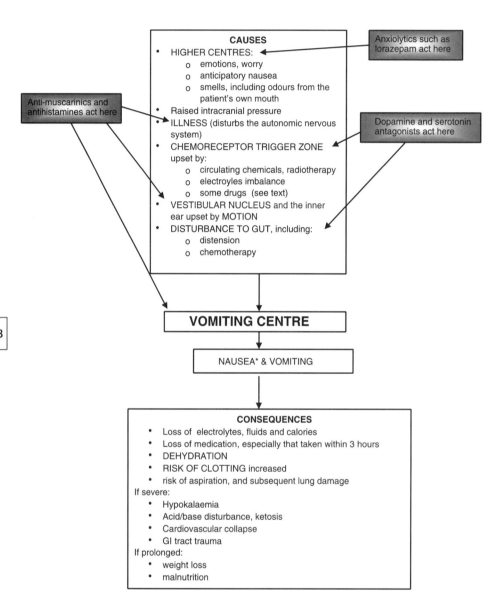

CAUSES
- HIGHER CENTRES:
  - o emotions, worry
  - o anticipatory nausea
  - o smells, including odours from the patient's own mouth
- Raised intracranial pressure
- ILLNESS (disturbs the autonomic nervous system)
- CHEMORECEPTOR TRIGGER ZONE upset by:
  - o circulating chemicals, radiotherapy
  - o electroyles imbalance
  - o some drugs (see text)
- VESTIBULAR NUCLEUS and the inner ear upset by MOTION
- DISTURBANCE TO GUT, including:
  - o distension
  - o chemotherapy

Anxiolytics such as lorazepam act here

Anti-muscarinics and antihistamines act here

Dopamine and serotonin antagonists act here

VOMITING CENTRE

NAUSEA* & VOMITING

CONSEQUENCES
- Loss of electrolytes, fluids and calories
- Loss of medication, especially that taken within 3 hours
- DEHYDRATION
- RISK OF CLOTTING increased
- risk of aspiration, and subsequent lung damage

If severe:
- Hypokalaemia
- Acid/base disturbance, ketosis
- Cardiovascular collapse
- GI tract trauma

If prolonged:
- weight loss
- malnutrition

*Nausea is the conscious recognition of subconscious excitation of the bilateral vomiting centres in the brainstem (Guyton & Hall 2000 p.769).

Figure 12.1   Causes and consequences of vomiting

Table 12.1 Indications for anti-emetics

Surgery	Most anti-emetics can be prescribed. Cyclizine may be sufficient. Granisetron may be reserved for vulnerable individuals or when other drugs have failed.
Chemotherapy and radiotherapy Low risk of emesis High risk of emesis Delayed emesis Anticipatory nausea	Domperidone or metoclopramide. $5HT_3$-antagonists, with dexamethasone or aprepitant, if necessary. Dexamethasone and metoclopramide or prochlorperazine or $5HT_3$-antagonists. Lorazepam, an anxiolytic.
Palliative care Hypercalcaemia, renal failure Bowel obstruction Excessive intestinal secretions Excessive respiratory tract secretions **Opioid therapy** Emesis may subside in four to five days, allowing withdrawal of anti-emetics	Haloperidol. Cyclizine. Octreotide. Hyoscine hydrobromide. Metoclopramide or haloperidol. Levomepromazine may be substituted for drug combinations. It is also sedative, anxiolytic and analgesic (BNF 2007).
Motion sickness $5HT_3$-antagonists, metoclopramide, domperidone and phenothiazines are ineffective	Hyoscine hydrobromide. Sedating anti-histamines, for example promethazine, are slightly less effective but cause less discomfort. Cyclizine should be offered to patients travelling in connection with anti-cancer treatment.
Gastrointestinal conditions such as, stress-induced gastric paresis/stasis and non-ulcer dyspepsia	Metoclopramide or domperidone restore peristalsis.
Migraine Administered at the onset of acute attack	Metoclopramide or domperidone overcome gastric stasis. To hasten absorption, or if vomiting is a problem, prochlorperazine can be administered as buccal tablets, placed between lips and gums.
Pregnancy First trimester, if severe. If symptoms do not resolve in 24–48 hours, seek medical advice.	Short-term treatment with an antihistamine, for example, promethazine, may help (Jordan 2002b).
Emergency hormonal contraception (associated nausea)	Domperidone.

Administration

◆ **Metoclopramide** is administered orally (tablets, liquid, oral solution or syrup), or by injection. Maximum dose depends on body weight, but may be increased during cancer treatments. Discoloured solutions should not be used. Effects begin 30 minutes to 1 hour after oral administration and last 1–3 hours. Emesis should be relieved in 10–15 minutes after intramuscular administration (usually into thigh, Figure 21.1) or 1–3 minutes after intravenous administration. Modified release preparations may not be bioequivalent to standard formulations.

◆ **Domperidone** is poorly absorbed (10–17%) and therefore acts mainly in the gut.

◆ **Hyoscine hydrobromide** may be administered orally, 30 minutes before start of a journey, or as a transdermal patch applied to hairless skin behind ear five to six hours before the journey.

◆ **5HT$_3$-antagonists** are administered an hour before chemotherapy. Effects last about 24 hours. Oral administration may be most effective.

Local reactions may occur when cyclizine, metoclopramide, levomepromazine are used in syringe drivers. Rectal administration is associated with irritation and erratic absorption (Box 1.2).

 Adverse effects: ANTI-MUSCARINICS and ANTIHISTAMINES

◆ **Drying of secretions**

◆ **Slowing of smooth muscle in gut, genito-urinary system and eye**

◆ **Quickening of the heart**
  Acetylcholine is the key neurotransmitter of the parasympathetic nervous system. Its muscarinic actions are blocked by: phenothiazines, prochlorperazine, hyoscine, procyclidine, orphenadrine, oxybutinin (for incontinence), antihistamines (above), (less commonly by haloperidol or metoclopramide), and the inhaled bronchodilators ipratropium and tiotropium. As a result, the body can no longer increase secretions, activate the smooth muscle of the gut and genito-urinary system, constrict the pupil or control the flow of acqueous humour in the eye, and slow the heart rate.

◆ **Neurological**
  Histamine and acetylcholine maintain arousal and awareness. Blocking their actions may cause sedation, confusion or hallucinations.

Adverse effects: implications for practice: ANTI-MUSCARINICS and ANTIHISTAMINES:

The importance of the adverse effects depends on the circumstances, and duration of therapy. (Most problems are dose-related.)

Problem	Suggestions for Prevention and Management
Drying of secretions	
Dry mouth, leading to: ◆ discomfort ◆ halitosis ◆ mouth ulcers ◆ discomfort from dentures	Advise on dental hygiene. Ensure prompt mouth care. Offer ice cubes and sips of water. Mouthwash may help. Check for oral thrush.

◆ dental caries with long-term use Also occurs with most other anti-emetics	Be aware that GTN sprays may be ineffective.
Drying of bronchial secretions. This increases risk of chest infections	Advise cessation of smoking. Encourage regular deep breathing. Maintain adequate hydration. Position and turn patients, if appropriate. Monitor lung bases and temperature for signs of chest infection, if appropriate.
Risk of middle ear infections. Movement of cilia of middle ear inhibited	If patient has an upper respiratory tract infection, if possible seek alternative therapy (Aronson 2006).
Dry skin, predisposing to pressure sores	Check pressure areas. Assess need for emollients.
Reduced ability to sweat	Avoid high environmental temperatures. Advise patient to seek help if fever develops.
Dry eyes	Advise patient to protect eyes from wind. Artificial tears if required. Recommend removal of contact lenses.
Gastrointestinal tract	
Gastric stasis and emesis	Monitor intake with long-term use. (See bronchodilators.)
Constipation	Monitor bowel movements if used for more than a few days. (See laxatives.)
Bladder	
Retention of urine, with overflow, particularly if prostate gland is enlarged	Monitor urine output. Check continence and other symptoms of urinary tract infection with long-term use. Inquire regarding constipation.
Vision	
Blurred vision Anti-muscarinics dilate the pupil, impairing the ability to focus on close work, reading, television or driving	Advise that this usually subsides within a few days. Caution if driving.
Photophobia The pupil cannot constrict, which causes eye pain in bright light	Ensure patient is not discomforted by direct exposure to bright lights or sunlight (Karch 2006).

101

Glaucoma (rare). In vulnerable people, drainage of the aqueous humour from the anterior chamber of the eye is impeded, allowing build-up of intra-ocular pressure	Report vision changes to prescriber. For long-term use, see antipsychotics.
Cardiovascular system	
Tachycardia may lead to heart failure or a cardiac event	Monitor pulse regularly. Report if outside range 55–90bpm. Inquire regarding chest pain or increasing breathlessness.
Hypotension	Monitor BP (see diuretics). Maintain fluid balance records to: ♦ avoid fluid depletion. ♦ ensure prompt rehydration after vomiting or diarrhoea. Advise patients to: ♦ change position slowly ♦ report any dizziness ♦ drink clear fluids.
Neurological	
Drowsiness. May abate after 2–3 days. Problem may return on withdrawal (Can also occur with metoclopramide)	Warn patients of this problem and its intensification if alcohol is co-administered. Advise regarding driving.
Confusion, impaired short-term memory, irritability, agitation, tremor, insomnia, nightmares, hallucinations, even psychosis (mainly in older patients)	Seek alternative anti-emetic. Avoid prolonged use or high doses.
Seizures (rare)	Close observation of children with a history of seizures.
Dependence	Discuss with prescriber.

Adverse effects:

DOPAMINE ANTAGONISTS: Dopamine is an important neurotransmitter in the control of posture and movement. Its actions are blocked by metoclopramide, prochlorperazine, phenothiazines, haloperidol, and cinnarizine in older people. These problems may be less likely with domperidone. They are rare with ondansetron and antihistamines. No reports with other $5HT_3$-antagonists, to date. For drowsiness, changes in heart rate, see anti-muscarinics, above.

Adverse effects: implications for practice: DOPAMINE ANTAGONISTS

Problem	Suggestions for Prevention and Management
Posture and movement disorders (see antipsychotics)	
Acute dystonia: abnormal facial spasms and body movements, including oculogyric crisis, or myoclonus (glossary), within 36 hours of administration, particularly young or very old patients	Remain with patient. Be prepared to administer procyclidine 5–10mg im or iv. Observe for any obstruction of the airway.
Restlessness, akathisia	Observe for abnormal 'hand-wringing' movements. Administer intravenous injections slowly.
Parkinsonian symptoms (tremor and slowed movements), swallowing difficulties, slurred speech after one to two weeks **Tardive dyskinesia if used for weeks or months**	Observe for abnormal movements or stiffness. Particular care with long-term therapy. Discuss alternative therapy, with prescriber.
Endocrine disturbance: Prolactin secretion is increased, with prolonged use.	
Gynaecomastia, menstrual disturbance	If discomfort occurs, seek alternative therapy.

Neuroleptic malignant syndrome is a rare adverse effect (see antipsychotics).

103

Adverse effects:

5HT$_3$-ANTAGONISTS/SEROTONIN ANTAGONISTS: Serotonin controls the contraction of the smooth muscle of the blood vessels. It constricts most blood vessels, but dilates blood vessels in the heart and skeletal muscle. Serotonin can change blood pressure by acting on the blood vessels or the nervous system. It also affects the excitability of nervous and conducting tissue (Katzung & Julius 2001).

Adverse effects: implications for practice: 5HT$_3$-ANTAGONISTS/ SEROTONIN ANTAGONISTS

Problem	Suggestions for Prevention and Management
Flushing, dizziness and headache are a result of vasodilation	Reassure. Simple analgesia (paracetamol).
Blood pressure changes	Monitor BP.
Cardiac dysrhythmias, including long QT interval (glossary) Problems can occur with intravenous administration in acute settings (rare, but serious) Dolasetron causes bradycardia	Ensure potassium concentration remains within normal limits. Administer intravenous preparations slowly. Monitor pulse. Be alert for symptoms such as palpitations, chest pain. Arrange ECG if concerned.
Sleepiness, weakness, anorexia Insomnia also reported	It may be appropriate to monitor food intake.
Seizures	Close observation of patients with history of seizures or receiving anti-epileptic drugs.

Adverse effects: implications for practice: MOST ANTI-EMETICS

Most anti-emetics can alter bowel movement, because motility of the GI tract depends on the neurotransmitters that control emesis.

Problem	Suggestions for Prevention and Management
Gastrointestinal problems	
Constipation after 2–3 days' use (women may be more vulnerable when using 5HT$_3$-antagonists (Viramontes et al. 2001))	Long-term therapy, see antipsychotics.
Worsening of bowel obstruction	Monitor bowel activity. Check bowel sounds.
Worsening of haemorrhoids, diverticular disease and heartburn	If appropriate, encourage adequate fluid intake, high fibre diet. Be prepared to administer appropriate laxative or gastric acid suppressant.
Diarrhoea (particularly domperidone, metoclopramide)	Ensure unimpeded access to bathroom. Monitor and replace electrolytes and fluids, as needed. Monitor BP and postural hypotension.
Hiccup (5HT$_3$-antagonists only)	Discuss alternative anti-emetic, with prescriber.
Therapeutic failure	
Vomiting continues	Consider all causes of emesis (Figure 12.1), and make patient as comfortable as possible. Discuss with prescriber, the use of additional anti-emetics, such as corticosteroids or anxiolytics, such as lorazepam.

Hypersensitivity response, including liver impairment, rashes, photosensitivity, bronchospasm, bone marrow suppression, are rare.

Cautions and contra-indications:

◆ Emesis may be symptomatic of life-threatening conditions, for example raised intra-cranial pressure, diabetic keto-acidosis. The urgent diagnosis of such conditions may be hindered by anti-emetics.

◆ Before anti-emetics are administered, the underlying problem should be corrected if possible: for example, infection, constipation, renal failure, chronic cough, disorders of the inner ear and electrolyte or thyroid imbalance.

◆ Drug-induced emesis is sometimes best managed by dosage reduction (see list above). If body weight is decreasing, as may occur in palliative care, a pre-existing regimen may induce emesis for the first time.

- **Metoclopramide and domperidone** increase gut motility and are contra-indicated if the gut is obstructed or traumatised. Avoid metoclopramide within three to four days of a surgical anastomosis.

- **Prochlorperazine, hyoscine, anti-muscarinics and antihistamines** are used very cautiously, if at all, for patients with histories of closed-angle glaucoma (also family history), prostatic hyperthrophy, urinary retention, bowel obstruction, liver impairment or epilepsy. If a patient has a fever or is in a hot environment, administration of any anti-muscarinic may increase body temperature.

- **Syringe drivers**: avoid prochlorperazine and chlorpromazine (high risk of painful skin reactions).

- **Parkinson's disease**: cyclizine is suitable. All dopamine antagonists (metoclopramide, prochlorperazine, haloperidol) worsen Parkinson's disease. Domperidone may be administered with caution.

- **Cardiac dysrhythmias** (or relevant history): dolasetron, tropisetron and antipsychotics are used cautiously, if at all.

- **Liver or kidney impairment, older adults**: doses of most anti-emetics are reduced.

- **Children/young people** may be more sensitive to certain adverse effects, including sedation, acute dystonic reactions. Doses are calculated according to body weight, which should be recorded on the drug chart in kilograms. Administration of metoclopramide to people <20 is restricted (BNF 2007).

- **Porphyria** (glossary): avoid metoclopramide, antihistamines.

- Antihistamines block responses to skin prick tests for allergy, and should not be administered for 1 week before testing.

Interactions (summary):
Combining anti-emetics usually increases the incidence of adverse effects. Intravenous metoclopramide and $5HT_3$-antagonists administered together are more likely to cause cardiac disturbances. Co-administration of drugs with opposing actions on the gut is unlikely to relieve emesis, for example metoclopramide or domperidone plus cyclizine or prochlorperazine. However, dexametasone enhances the effects of $5HT_3$-antagonists and dopamine antagonists. Adverse effects are more likely if drugs with similar actions are co-administered (Table 12.2).

Table 12.2 Adverse effects associated with co-administration

Sedatives For example, opioids, anxiolytics, phenothiazines, alcohol, lithium, anti-epileptics, some herbal remedies, including valerian, *kava kava*	+ Most anti-emetics	→ Increased sedation, impaired driving skills
Antipsychotics fluoxetine, paroxetine or lithium	+ Any dopamine antagonist	→ Increased risk of involuntary movements

ANTI-EMETICS

Drugs with antimuscarinic actions e.g. antihistamines, antipsychotics, tricyclic antidepressants, drugs for incontinence e.g. oxybutinin, muscle relaxants e.g. baclofen, some herbal remedies e.g. *Atropa belladonna*	+ Cyclizine, hyoscine, promethazine, prochlorperazine, procyclidine	→ Dry mouth Increased risk of constipation, urine retention, confusion or (rarely) glaucoma

Metoclopramide increases the rate of absorption of many drugs, including alcohol, morphine, ciclosporin and paracetamol, and enhances actions of suxamethonium. This is attributed to acceleration of gastric emptying. It also increases the risk of kidney damage with cisplatin.

Antimuscarinics reduce absorption of levodopa or haloperidol.

In patients with severe heart failure receiving opioids, administration of **cyclizine** may induce severe breathlessness.

Anti-emetics are often combined with diamorphine in **syringe drivers**. However, under certain conditions, such as high concentrations, they are incompatible, causing the formation of visible solid precipitates, see BNF 'Prescribing in palliative care' for details.

Contributor

David Gallimore BSc, MSc, RGN, is tutor in adult nursing, School of Health Science, University of Wales, Swansea

13 Opioid analgesics

Opioid analgesics relieve pain caused by tissue damage.

Opioids include: morphine, diamorphine, pethidine/meperidine, meptazinol, dihydro-codeine(df118), codeine, buprenorphine, tramadol, fentanyl, remifentanil, methadone, and the "morphine antagonist or blocker", naloxone.

Actions: Opioids are analgesic and anxiolytic: this dual action is helpful in some clinical situations. They are similar to endorphins and enkephalins, which are the body's natural mood changers and analgesics in times of stress. They interact with dopamine in the areas of the brain associated with 'reward'. Prescribed opioids act on the different types of opioid receptors of the spinal cord, brain stem, cerebral cortex and smooth muscle. Generally, opioids (endogenous and pharmacological) depress the activity of nerve or smooth muscle cells and have a calming effect. Sometimes, sedation, mental detachment or euphoria are the predominant effects, and the patient may be able to tolerate pain, while still perceiving the sensation.

Opioids regulate the endocrine, gastrointestinal, autonomic and immune systems, and may trigger histamine release. They also act directly on the neurones of the chemoreceptor trigger zone, which activates the vomiting centre (anti-emetics Figure 12.1).

Indications:

◆ pain and trauma.
◆ severe pain in palliative care.
◆ surgery.
◆ myocardial infarction: slow intravenous diamorphine.
◆ acute pulmonary oedema: slow intravenous diamorphine.
◆ analgesia and suppression of respiratory activity in patients receiving intensive care and assisted ventilation.
◆ cough suppression in terminal care.

Specialists sometimes prescribe opioids for chronic non-malignant pain (Gutstein & Akil 2006). Such patients may need advice regarding driving.

Administration: Where pain is anticipated opioids should be administered regularly. If pain has built-up, the dose needed to achieve analgesia may induce sedation. Less drug is needed to prevent pain than to relieve it. Patients who are older, debilitated, malnourished, or have impaired renal or hepatic function require lower or less frequent doses.

Morphine. Oral morphine is often the opioid of choice for pain control in palliative care. The proportion absorbed is increased by food and varies between individuals. Extra doses may be needed for painful procedures, such as dressing changes; these should be administered 30 minutes before the procedure. Morphine can be administered as modified release capsules, which can be opened and added to soft food and swallowed without chewing (BNF 2007 p. 229, Box 1.1).

Buprenorphine can be administered orally, sublingually, transdermally or by injection. Different brands of transdermal patches deliver different doses. Times taken to achieve analgesia and duration of action also differ. Buprenorphine may cause withdrawal reactions a few days after discontinuation and in patients accustomed to opioid use. It is also prescribed in substance misuse teams.

Codeine, dihydrocodeine and dextropropoxyphene are included in some compound preparations with paracetamol. At these low doses, they often provide very little analgesia, but can cause unpleasant side effects: codeine is very constipating and dihydrocodeine causes nausea, particularly in older people.

Diamorphine/heroin is highly lipid-soluble therefore:

◆ It readily crosses the blood-brain barrier and rapidly relieves pain and distress.

◆ Enough diamorphine for 24 hours can be placed in small patient-controlled analgesia devices or syringe drivers. Low volume subcutaneous infusions cause less oedema and induration at the syringe driver site (Fonzo-Christe *et al.* 2005).

Fentanyl is twice as lipid-soluble as diamorphine. It can be absorbed through the lining of the mouth. It acts within 5 minutes and lasts 80–90 minutes. Lozenges may be administered 5 minutes before wound dressings or for breakthrough pain. Single and multiple doses of fentanyl buccal tablets may not be bioequivalent (glossary) (Darwish *et al.* 2006).

In palliative care, skin patches may offer convenient alternatives to syringe drivers (Box 13.1). Patches are changed every 72 hours. The prolonged action of transdermal fentanyl means that dose titration may be difficult. The full effects of a patch will not be experienced for 24 hours, and monitoring should be continued for 24 hours after removal.

Box 13.1 Transdermal administration of medications

Gloves are worn when handling patches and skin preparations (Smith *et al.* 2008). Gloves are not impermeable, and hand washing is important (Pratt *et al.* 2007). Ensure that patches are applied to:

◆ Hairless, unshaved areas. Shaving disrupts hair follicles, increasing absorption.

◆ Dry skin, free of irritants, including soap.

◆ Upper arms, chest or back (usually). The upper back is often the best site for patients who may be confused or inclined to interfere with the patch. The thin skin behind the ear is a popular site for hyoscine patches.

◆ Sites which have not been used for several days, longer if advised by manufacturers (some buprenorphine patches, should not be re-applied for 3 weeks (BNF 2007)).

Advise that:

◆ Palm pressure for 30 seconds should ensure closure of patch edges.

◆ On removal, patches should be folded. Used patches contain sufficient medication to warrant disposal in 'biohazard' containers, rather than general waste (Smith *et al.* 2008).

- ◆ Increased absorption may occur if the patient or patch becomes hot, due to a fever, hot bath, electric blanket or environmental conditions.
- ◆ Inflammation may occur at the patch site. This should be reported. Particular care over possible delayed reactions to buprenorphine patches.
- ◆ Should a patch fall off, medication should be removed from the skin and a new patch may be applied on a new site.

Hydromorphone capsules may be swallowed whole or the contents sprinkled onto food. Modified release capsules and the 4-hourly capsules contain different quantities of the drug.

Pethidine/meperidine accumulates with prolonged administration. To avoid irritation, scarring or fibrosis at injection sites, ensure sites are documented and not re-used.

Tramadol. In addition to its opioid actions, tramadol enhances the actions of serotonin and noradrenaline/norepinephrine. Therefore, it has additional adverse effects, such as hypertension, diarrhoea, confusion.

Naloxone reverses the effects of other opioids, including: respiratory depression, sedation, itching, myoclonus (glossary) and analgesia. The half-life (glossary) and duration of action of naloxone are much shorter than those of morphine, diamorphine, pethidine, fentanyl and other opioids (1 hour *versus* 2–5 hours). Therefore, the effects of naloxone wear off before those of the other opioid, allowing problems to re-emerge. Following administration, close observation is required to identify any recurrence of respiratory depression.

Adverse effects:

- ◆ **Central nervous system depression and sedation.** Opioids act directly on the respiratory centre in the brain stem to depress respiration. They reduce the sensitivity of the respiratory centre to carbon dioxide, thus reducing the normal drive to respiration. Rate, depth and regularity of respirations are decreased, reducing the amount of air reaching the alveoli, and oxygenation of the body. Depression of the carbon dioxide respiratory drive means that the patient's breathing depends on the hypoxic respiratory drive. Administration of a high concentration of oxygen to a patient whose respirations are depressed due to opioids can remove the remaining respiratory drive and precipitate a sudden respiratory arrest. This may be difficult to reverse, due to a sharp rise in carbon dioxide concentration (Gutstein & Akil 2006). Respiratory problems are compounded by the depression of the cough reflex and inhibition of the cilia lining the respiratory tract. These problems may continue after pain relief has ceased. More rarely, the cardiovascular centres in the brain stem are depressed.
- ◆ **Stimulation of excitable tissues.** Opioids reduce the availability of the neurotransmitter responsible for inhibiting the nervous system, GABA. This can cause excitability.
- ◆ **Gastrointestinal disturbances.** Opioids act on the smooth muscle of the gut to inhibit peristalsis, causing gastric stasis, delayed transit and constipation. At the same time, they intensify sphincter contractions and the segmental contractions of the gut or the common bile duct. This can cause spasms and colic.
- ◆ **Genito-urinary disturbances.** Opioids act in the hypothalamus to increase secretion

of prolactin and reduce secretion of luteinizing hormone. This reduces secretion of testosterone and inhibits ovulation. Opioids can cause spasm of the urethral sphincter.

◆ **Impaired immunity.** Opioids cause histamine release, unrelated to hypersensitivity responses. There are opioid receptors on the cells of the immune system. Both pain and opioids suppress the immune system. Overall, opioids boost the immune system by relieving pain (Gutstein & Akil 2006).

Adverse effects: implications for practice: OPIOIDS

The commonest side effects of opioids are nausea, vomiting, constipation, drowsiness. Large doses produce respiratory depression and hypotension.

Potential Problem	Suggestions for Prevention and Management
Central nervous system depression	
Respiratory depression **Particularly older people and children** **Delayed reactions are possible, up to 11 hours, particularly with intrathecal or epidural administration**	Assess respiratory rate, depth and rhythm before and during therapy: particularly at 5–10 minutes after intravenous and 30–90 minutes after intra-muscular administration of morphine. Continue monitoring up to 23 hours after discontinuation. If respiratory rate falls below 12/minute (adults) or breathing is unduly shallow or irregular, withhold drug and contact prescriber. Check oxygenation with pulse oximeter (always in children (Aronson 2006)). Ensure naloxone is available to reverse respiratory depression, if necessary. Administer naloxone cautiously if a patient is at risk of cardiac dysrhythmia. Expect to administer at least two doses of naloxone.
Carbon dioxide retention **Respiratory arrest, due to loss of carbon dioxide respiratory drive**	Avoid administration of high dose oxygen to patients whose respirations are depressed due to opioids.
Risk of chest infection **Due to cough suppression and paralysis of respiratory cilia, secretions are not cleared from the airways**	Ensure patient is hydrated. Dessicated mucus is more likely to form plugs and block the airways. Position and turn patient to reduce risk of chest infection. Monitor respirations. Encourage regular deep breathing. Advise cessation of smoking. Monitor lung bases and temperature for signs of chest infection, if appropriate.
Bronchospasm **Histamine release causes bronchoconstriction and**	Opioids are not administered during asthma attacks.

may occasionally precipitate an asthma attack	
Hypotension, orthostatic hypotension **Risk of falling, particularly if patient is dehydrated.**	Careful monitoring on commencing infusions. Care when moving patients from supine to head-up positions. Advise patients to mobilise slowly and report any dizziness. Monitor BP and heart rate lying and sitting. Fluid balance. Ensure intravenous fluids available to correct hypovolaemia and hypotension.
Bradycardia	Check heart rate During infusions, ensure atropine is available to reverse bradycardia if necessary.
Sedation **Cognitive impairment**	Monitor consciousness/drowsiness. Avoid other sedatives. Driving/ skilled tasks may be affected. Patients using patches who develop a fever should be monitored for sedation and changes in vital signs, and prescribers informed.
Aspiration of gastric contents associated with depression of gag reflex	Minimise sedation and nausea. Put the patient in the recovery position should vomiting occur.
Poor thermoregulation	Record temperature carefully, otherwise a fever could be overlooked.
Stimulation of excitable tissues	
Hallucinations, disturbed sleep, shadows in peripheral vision	Warn patients or carers. Offer reassurance and explanation. Encourage fluids: these problems are more likely if the patient is dehydrated (Aronson 2006).
Convulsions, particularly: children, high doses, tramadol, repeated doses of pethidine	Observe for signs of cerebral irritability. Ensure naloxone is available. Anticonvulsants may not be effective (Gutstein & Akil 2006).
Euphoria/dysphoria	Tolerance may develop within two to three days. Codeine is the least problematic opioid.
Myoclonus and muscular rigidity, which may affect the chest wall (particularly high doses, pethidine, bolus fentanyl)	Administer intravenous injections slowly. Ensure respiration is not compromised during anaesthesia with fentanyl or related drugs due to rigidity of chest wall. Check oxygenation Ensure naloxone is available. Discuss, with prescriber, possibility of excessive dose.

Pupil constriction (not pethidine) Smooth muscle of the iris is constricted by excitation of the parasympathetic nerve	Avoid opioids when neurological observations are needed e.g. after head injury.
Gastrointestinal disturbances	
Nausea, vomiting or gastric reflux (about 67% of patients affected) (See anti-emetics)	Provide support to reduce anxiety, fear and pain. Avoid sudden movements, particularly of the head. Extra care during transfers. Allow extra time for transfers. Advise patients that resting decreases nausea. Administer anti-emetics, as requested, for 2–3 days and advise the patient that tolerance may develop. Monitor food intake and nutrition status.
Constipation	If prescription is likely to exceed five days administer laxatives with the first dose of opioid. (See laxatives) No tolerance develops: as dose increases, so does constipation. Auscultate for bowel sounds.
Constriction of anal sphincter	Anticipate difficulties with rectal administration of medication, if the sphincter is tight and the rectum is full.
Obstruction	Monitor bowel evacuations. Recognise colicky abdominal pain as an early sign of bowel obstruction.
Biliary colic (acute abdominal pain)	Be aware that opioids may worsen biliary colic and cause a rise in serum amylase. Ensure nitrates or atropine are available, should the prescriber request these.
Dry mouth	Assist with oral hygiene. Use moist oral swabs in patients with dysphagia.
Genito-urinary system	
Menstrual irregularities	Fertility is impaired by long-term use of many opioids, but not methadone. Ensure clients who are switching from heroin to methadone receive adequate advice on contraception.
Reduced testosterone secretion (long-term use only)	Discuss, with prescriber, effects on bone health.
Urine retention **Opioids cause contraction of the urethral sphincter**	Monitor urine output. Be prepared to undertake bladder scan to assess retention.

Reduced renal perfusion If blood pressure is lowered, blood may be diverted away from the kidneys	Urine output should be monitored to exclude oliguria and retention of urine. Output should be at least 600mls/day.

Immune system

Pruritus, rashes, urticaria, flushing (particularly at injection or patch sites and on the face), due to histamine release	Ensure coolant gels are available. Antihistamines may not relieve itching. Low doses of naloxone or ondansetron may be effective. Avoid epidural administration of morphine.
Increased infections with long-term use	Monitor patients for signs of infection.
Reactivation of *Herpes simplex* infections	Observe patients following epidural administration. Discuss prescription of topical treatments, with prescriber.

Therapeutic failure

Pain fails to respond	Consider that pain may be due to damaged nerves (neuropathic pain). Opioids are of little help in this type of pain. Consider adequacy of dose, particularly if the patient has a history of recreational drug use. Be prepared to increase the dose to accommodate tolerance (even within 24 hours) or symptom progression. Some patients require up to 500mgs morphine daily (BNF 2007). If the drug has been administered intra-muscularly, check that the patient is not in shock or heart failure. Poor circulation causes delayed absorption. Discuss alternative opioid, with prescriber. Some patients who derive no benefit or experience intolerable adverse effects from one opioid will be helped by another.
Pain intensifies when opioid has worn off	Ensure patient can operate any patient controlled device. If analgesia is prescribed 'as needed', ensure patients understand the need to contact staff at the first sensation of pain.
Withdrawal symptoms Lacrimation, runny nose, sweating, yawning start 8–12 hours after last dose, followed by irritability, insomnia, weakness, anxiety, depression, anrexia, emesis, diarrhoea, dehydration, cramps, fever peaking at about 24–48 hours	Ensure that dose and preparation changes are undertaken gradually. Observe patient for emergence of any rebound pain and other symptoms on withdrawal, dose reduction or regimen change. Dose reductions of 10–20% every other day should prevent withdrawal symptoms (Gutstein & Akil 2006).

Rare adverse effects reported with epidural, intrathecal or intravenous administration include: vertigo, nystagmus (glossary), blurred vision, catatonia, epidural fibrosis, cough, aggression. Additional adverse effects may occur in those over-using non-prescription opioids, including lung damage, renal failure, nervous system damage, fetotoxicity.

Cautions and contra-indications:

◆ Increased intra-cranial pressure (stroke, head injury). Opioids may increase intra-cranial pressure and obscure vital signs/pupil reflexes.

◆ Decreased respiratory reserve, including obesity and kyphosis; contra-indicated if $p\text{CO}_2$ (carbon dioxide partial pressure or concentration) is increased.

◆ Pregnancy and breastfeeding (Jordan 2002b).

◆ Dependence (unimportant in palliative care).

◆ Known allergy to opioids.

◆ Renal insufficiency.

◆ Dextropropoxyphene should be avoided where overdose is possible as it induces heart failure.

◆ Neonates and premature babies require proportionately lower doses, due to the high permeability of the blood-brain barrier. Fentanyl may cause jaundice.

Conditions which may be worsened include:

◆ asthma.

◆ acute alcohol intoxication.

◆ liver failure.

◆ convulsive disorders (particularly tramadol, pethidine).

◆ biliary colic, pancreatitis.

◆ conditions where there is a possibility of paralytic ileus.

◆ pre-existing hypotension, for example due to haemorrhage.

◆ hypothyroidism or Addison's disease.

◆ phaeochromocytoma (glossary).

◆ enlarged prostate.

◆ myasthenia gravis.

Opioids are no longer recommended for:

◆ cough suppression in children.

◆ management of diarrhoea.

115

Interactions (summary):

Hypotension, sedation and respiratory depression may be intensified by: alcohol, antihistamines, barbiturates, anaesthetics (nitrous oxide), benzodiazepines, metoclopramide, phenothiazines, tricyclic antidepressants, and other non-opioid sedatives. Protease inhibitors, cimetidine, and occasionally ranitidine, may have this effect.

Central nervous system toxicity may occur if: pethidine (possibly also fentanyl and dextropropoxyphene) are administered within two weeks of any MAOI (including moclobemide and (possibly) linezolid) or selegiline or rasagiline (for Parkinson's); tramadol is co-administered with most antidepressants; dextromethorphan is co-administered with memantine (for dementia).

Myoclonus is more likely with co-administration of: chlorpromazine, haloperidol, amitriptyline and some NSAIDs (but not diclofenac).

Drying of secretions, and therefore need for mouth care, is intensified by co-administration of hyoscine, cyclizine or related drugs, see anti-emetics.

Oestrogens (including oral contraceptives), phenytoin, carbamazepine and rifampicin decrease the effectiveness of some opioids. Phenytoin increases the risk of toxicity with pethidine. Antiviral and antifungal drugs may affect opioid concentrations.

Dextropropoxyphene intensifies the effects of warfarin and carbamazepine.

Opioid-induced gastric stasis may delay or impair absorption of other drugs, for example paracetamol.

Drugs are often mixed in **syringe drivers**, but compatibilities may be complicated (see BNF).

Contributor

Jeanette Hewitt RMN, RGN, RNT, BSc (Hons), PGCE, PGCertCouns. Lecturer, School of Health Sciences, Swansea University

14 Antiepileptic drugs: focus on carbamazepine and valproate

Antiepileptic drugs are prescribed to eliminate, minimise or control seizures, while avoiding serious adverse drug reactions.

Actions: Antiepileptic drugs (listed below) reduce the activity of neurones in the central nervous system. This is achieved by either direct action on the neurones or augmenting the inhibitory neurotransmitter, gamma-aminobutyric acid (GABA). While this reduces the number of seizures, it also suppresses the normal functions of the CNS. This may lead to sedation, inco-ordination or even depression of vital signs.

Each neurone's (nerve cell's) activity depends on the balance between positive and negative ions entering the cell (Figure 14.1). This balance may be disturbed in epilepsy. Epilepsy and over-activity (or repetitive firing) of neurones are associated with excess sodium ion or calcium ion entry. Entry of these ions is blocked by some antiepileptics (carbamazepine, phenytoin, lamotrigine). Since these ions are required by many cells, these drugs affect most body systems. Other drugs restore the balance or 'calm down' the neurones by increasing the number of negative ions entering the cells. Benzodiazepines and barbiturates increase the number of negative chloride ions entering the neurones, by acting on the GABA

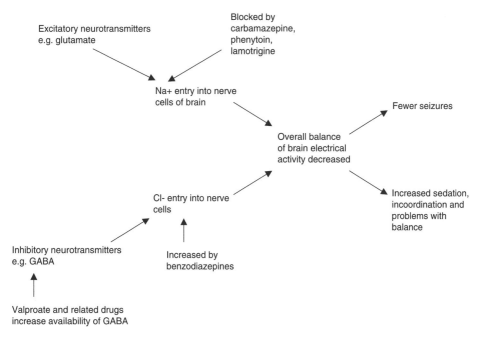

Figure 14.1 Actions of antiepileptic drugs

receptor. Other drugs (valproate, gabapentin) increase the amount of GABA, which inhibits the activity (or firing) of neurones by increasing the entry of negative chloride ions.

Indications and administration: Specialists select appropriate anti-epileptic agents, in accordance with type of epilepsy or pattern of seizures, and individuals' lifestyles or preferences. Where possible, epilepsy is controlled by a single drug (NICE 2004c). There is often a very narrow therapeutic range between seizures and sedation. For some people, even a delayed dose can allow seizure breakthrough.

◆ Carbamazepine: taken 2–3 times/day, with meals to reduce gastric irritation. Modified release preparations are taken 1–2 times/day. Concentration peaks 4–24 hours after ingestion. Dosage may need to be increased within the first few weeks' of therapy. For patients taking up to 1g/day, suppositories can be substituted for up to 7 days, but careful dose adjustments are needed, because suppositories are not bioequivalent (glossary) to oral medicines. Rectal irritation may occur. Oxcarbazepine is similar.

◆ Gabapentin: usually as adjunct treatment, 3 doses/day, 2 hours apart from antacids.

◆ Lamotrigine: taken once or twice each day. Only dispersible tablets can be chewed.

◆ Levetiracetam tablets are swallowed whole, twice daily.

◆ Phenytoin is taken 1–3 times/day with food and water to reduce gastric irritation. Mixing with food or enteral feeds is not advised. In status epilepticus intravenous fosphenytoin is an alternative.

◆ Tiagabine: 2–4 doses/day with food.

◆ Topiramate: broken tablets give a bitter taste – avoid. Swallow 'sprinkle capsules' immediately after adding to food.

◆ Valproate: taken 2–3 times/day, with food to reduce nausea. Modified release preparations taken once or twice daily. Maintain consistent relation to meals.

◆ Vigabatrin is prescribed on specialist advice (see vision, below).

◆ Benzodiazepines become less effective with regular use over 1–6 months. They are important in emergency treatment:

❖ Status epilepticus: usual management is intravenous lorazepam

❖ Recurrent seizures, premonitary stage:
  • diazepam as rectal solution, or
  • midazolam, as buccal liquid (Walker 2005), following training (NICE 2004c), intramuscular or intravenous injections (unlicensed).

Pregabelin and zonisamide have been introduced as adjunct therapy.

Barbiturates, ethosuximide, acetazolamide, corticosteroids, paraldehyde are occasionally prescribed.
Some antiepileptics are also prescribed for neuropathic pain (carbamazepine, gabapentin, valproate) and mood disorders (carbamazepine, valproate). In older patients, doses are lower and intravenous administration is slower.

Different brands and formulations may not be bioequivalent. Patients whose epilepsy is controlled may suffer recurrence of seizures if brands or formulations are interchanged (Chappell 1993). Seek advice from prescribers and/or pharmacists before undertaking any substitutions.

Adverse effects:

◆ **Nervous system** depression and dysfunction. Neuronal inhibition can affect all functions of the central nervous system, particularly those controlling balance. Both excitatory and inhibitory neurones may be depressed, resulting in either sedation or over-activity.

◆ **Alteration of body-image**
  ❖ Prolactin production may be increased by carbamazepine, phenytoin or poly-pharmacy (see antipsychotics).
  ❖ Valproate is associated with weight gain and secretion of excess androgens, which can affect the ovaries and the skin.
  ❖ Men taking carbamazepine may have reduced androgen secretion (Aronson 2006).

◆ The cardiovascular and gastrointestinal systems may also be affected.

◆ **Nutrition and electrolyte imbalance.** Some anti-epileptics speed-up metabolism, increasing the elimination of vital nutrients, such as folates and vitamin D.

Adverse effects: implications for practice: ANTIEPILEPTICS

Many adverse effects appear days or weeks after initiation of therapy. The full effects of valproate are not experienced for 3–4 days after initiation, and those of carbamazepine for 1–2 weeks. Doses are not usually incremented during these periods. Adverse events are particularly likely during illness or regimen change, including switching to chewable tablets.

Venous blood samples that may be required are summarised in Box 14.1.

Box 14.1   Measurements from venous blood samples

Valproate

◆ LFTs, pre-therapy, regularly for 6/12

◆ ammonia

◆ FBC, platelets, prothrombin and bleeding times – pre-therapy, follow up

◆ Fibrinogen

Carbamazepine or phenytoin

◆ FBC

◆ Electrolytes

◆ LFTs

◆ Vitamin D

◆ Calcium and alkaline phosphatase

Every 2–5 years (NICE 2004c) lipid profile is needed to assess cardiovascular risk.

Many of the problems below are common to most therapeutic regimens. Problems confined to certain drugs are indicated.

Potential Problem	Suggestions for Prevention and Management
Neurological	
Sedation, drowsiness, slurred speech, cognitive impairment, fatigue, confusion, poor concentration, headaches **Paraesthesia, muscle weakness** **Dizziness, unsteadiness/ataxia, incoordination**	Observe for drowsiness/tiredness. Monitor school performance and speech development. Inform patients that drowsiness will affect motor function and reaction time, at least initially. Driving may be affected. Monitor risk of falls in the elderly (Perucca *et al.* 2006). Discuss, with prescriber, possibilities of dividing the daily dose into smaller fractions or administration at bedtime. Check for nystagmus (jerky eye movements, glossary). This may be the first sign that doses are too high. Prescriber may request venous blood samples (particularly carbamazepine, Box 14.2). Some problems may subside within the first weeks.
Agitation, behaviour disturbance, hallucinations, depression, aggression, hyperactivity (psychoisis rarely) **Particular concern for clients with learning difficulties or previous history of mental illness. (vigabatrin, lamotrigine, gabapentin, levetiracetam)**	Monitor behaviour and school performance. Consider any possible association between disturbed behaviour and seizure frequency or withdrawal of medication. Request medication review.
Tremors, twitching (particularly valproate, about 9% clients) **Nervousness, insomnia, enuresis**	Monitor tremor and any impact on activities (see antipsychotics). Discuss prescription of slow-release preparations or dose reduction.
Posture and movement disorders, tics (valproate, ethosuximide, carbamazepine, lamotrigine, in high doses)	Report abnormal movements or changes in posture. For patients co-prescribed antipsychotic medication, complete recognised assessment instruments.
Hearing impairment **Valproate, possibly gabapentin, carbamazepine**	Report to prescriber if the patient experiences tinnitus or notices any change of pitch.
Fever (mainly topiramate)	Monitor patients, particularly children. Ensure that sweating is not impaired.

Vision	
Double or blurred vision possible with most antiepileptics	Discuss, with prescriber: ◆ possibility that the plasma concentration of antiepileptic is too high (Box 14.2) ◆ dividing the daily dose.
Visual field loss, vigabatrin (30% patients), tiagabine rarely	Arrange for eyes and visual fields to be tested pre-therapy and at 6-monthly intervals. This is difficult in young children. Advise patients to report any vision changes. Refer to ophthalmologist.
Myopia or glaucoma **Ethosuximide, topiramate** **Disturbance of colour vision, lens opacities carbamazepine**	Ensure that patients visit opticians regularly. Particular vigilance during first month of topiramate therapy.
Conjunctivitis, lamotrigine	Report to prescriber. This may be a hypersensitivity response.
Gastrointestinal disturbances are common	
Nausea, vomiting, anorexia (16% of those taking valproate) **Diarrhoea or constipation**	Taking new medication or increased doses with food may reduce nausea. This may subside in 2–3 weeks.
Dry, irritated mouth	Suggest regular water rinses. Valproate tablets: avoid chewing, taking with milk. Valproate syrup: avoid administering with carbonated drinks.
Alteration of body or self-image	
Coarsening of features, acne, hirsuitism, gynaecomastia, **Gum and lip hyperplasia. (Phenytoin, carbamazepine, ethosuximide, valproate)**	Consider impact of changes, and adherence to medication regimen. Scrupulous oral care. Liaise with dental hygienist and dentist experienced with this condition.
Hair loss **(Valproate 8%, carbamazepine)**	Hair regrowth with valproate may be curly. Loss more likely with higher plasma concentrations.
Weight gain **Valproate, vigabatrin, gabapentin, carbamazepine** **Anorexia/weight loss**	Monitor weight, pre-therapy and weekly. If weight changes, monitor diet. (see antipsychotics) Monitor growth in children.

Carbamazepine, topiramate, zonisamide, ethosuximide, lamotrigine, levetiracetam	
Reproduction: amenorrhoea, impaired fertility, polycystic ovaries in susceptible women. (valproate, carbamazepine, gabapentin) **Impotence, decreased libido (gabapentin, carbamazepine)** **Increased libido, vaginal bleeding (Ethosuximide)**	Discuss with nurse of the same gender. Refer to prescriber. Seek specialist advice. Prompt recognition of polycystic ovaries is helpful, as the condition may reverse on change of therapy (Aronson 2006).

Cardiovascular system

Cardiovascular or respiratory depression following intravenous administration for *status epilepticus*	Overdose and intravenous administration require monitoring of vital signs plus ECG, before, during and after infusions. Administer intravenous drugs slowly.
Bradycardia and heart block, changes in BP **Carbamazepine, oxcarbazepine**	Monitor vital signs and any dysrhythmias on initiation of therapy.
Oedema (valproate, carbamazepine, oxcarbazepine, gabapentin) **The nephrons' ability to excrete sodium may be reduced**	Monitor body weight to detect fluid retention, which may be associated with heart failure. Ask patients to report ankle oedema. Consider the risk of skin breakdown over lower legs and pressure areas.
Thromboembolism. **Carbamazepine, topiramate**	Ensure patients are not dehydrated. Assess cardiovascular risks.

Nutrition and electrolyte imbalance

Osteomalacia: fractures in adults: rickets and short stature in children	Monitor growth Encourage patient to eat foods high in calcium (dairy products), vitamin D (oily fish) (see corticosteroids). Discuss, with physician, arranging bone assessments, and any need for further protective measures (Aronson 2006).

Folate deficiency increases cardiovascular risks and causes anaemia (Carbamazepine, phenytoin, possibly lamotrigine)	Monitor full blood count (FBC) regularly. If folic acid is prescribed, phenytoin concentrations should be monitored (Baxter 2006).
Hyponatraemia and SIADH (see SSRIs, glossary) (Carbamazepine, oxcarbazepine, phenytoin)	Monitor sodium concentrations, particularly if older patients, or those with head injury, become confused or are co-prescribed diuretics or SSRIs.

Hypersensitivity responses and organ damage (chapter 21): Particular vigilance during first 8 weeks

Blood disorders/bone marrow suppression Platelet dysfunction and bleeding Anaemia Reduced white cell count Aplastic anaemia, rarely Lymph node enlargement (carbamazepine, phenytoin, lamotrigine)	Report any sore throats, mouth ulcers, fever, delayed healing, abnormal bruising or bleeding immediately. Check FBC and prothrombin time. FBC and coagulation tests advised for carbamazepine, ethosuximide, phenytoin, valproate and possibly lamotrigine, pre-therapy, pre-surgery and regularly. Ensure anaesthetic team is aware of medication. [Specialists will advise on the significance of abnormalities.]
Skin reactions, some very serious, can occur with all antiepileptics Particularly lamotrigine (0.8% children) and co-administration of valproate	Check temperature: fever may indicate a generalised reaction. Be prepared to increment doses gradually. Ask patients or parents to report any rash or flu-like symptoms immediately. Delay or mis-diagnosis may allow serious complications to develop.
Increased risk of sunburn Lamotrigine, carbamazepine	Advise covering skin with clothing and high factor/ high star sunscreen during exposure to sunlight. (see antipsychotics)

Organ damage

Renal impairment (chapter 21) Carbamazepine, ethosuximide, possibly gabapentin Kidney stones (topiramate, zonisamide) Urinary tract infection (gabapentin)	Pre-therapy and regular monitoring of plasma creatinine, urea and potassium and urine albumin/microalbumin concentrations. (Gabapentin can interfere with these urine tests.) Ensure patients remain well hydrated. Monitor urine, should frequency or dysuria develop.

123

Liver Impairment (Valproate, carbamazepine, ethosuximide, lamotrigine, phenytoin)	Report any light-coloured stools, vomiting, drowsiness, confusion or jaundice immediately. Monitor liver function and prothrombin time pre-therapy and monthly for 6 months (valproate) or regularly (carbamazepine) (Taylor *et al.* 2005).
Increased production of ammonia (valproate)	Elevated concentrations of liver enzymes should be reported, but prescribers may not discontinue medication.
Increased plasma concentrations of gamma-GT (Carbamazepine, phenytoin)	Be aware this does not indicate alcohol misuse.
Pancreatitis Valproate, gabapentin	If acute abdominal pain and vomiting develop, arrange venous blood samples to measure glucose and amylase concentrations.
Hypothyroidism Carbamazepine, phenytoin (rare)	If patients gain weight, become cold intolerant and lethargic, consider thyroid function tests.

Withdrawal

Abrupt withdrawal of medication	Discontinuation of therapy may induce seizures, even *status epilepticus,* or behaviour disturbance. Advise medi-alert identification.
Planned withdrawal: If no fits have occurred for 2–4 years, prescribers may gradually withdraw medication over 9–13 weeks or several months	Monitor patients for recurrence of seizures during withdrawal and for 12 months. Driving is not recommended during this time and for 6 months afterwards. Advise that, following a fit, the client will be banned from driving for 1 year (BNF 2007).

Therapeutic failure: The changes at cellular level (Figure 14.1) may be insufficient to bring about a clinical improvement

Not all epilepsy responds to medical management. Seizures can be controlled in some 50% patients, and reduced significantly in a further 25% (McNamara 2006)	**Acute care:** Keep oxygen and suction at bedside. Be prepared to administer emergency treatments (Taylor *et al.* 2005) **Prevention:** Assess **compliance.** Ask patients to take medication at equal intervals during the day. Doses should be neither omitted nor doubled-up. Warn patients that there may be a delay of several days between an omitted dose and a seizure. Record all seizures. Advise that seizures may be induced by: ◆ Abrupt discontinuation of antiepileptics ◆ Fever, infections, alcohol, substance misuse, sleep-deprivation, fatigue, stress, loud noise, hot baths or (in primary generalised epilepsy) flickering lights.

	◆ Overdose of antiepileptic medication. Help patients attend all appointments.
Loss of medication during vomiting	Ask patients to note the time of vomiting in relation to medication administration. Tablets taken up to 3 hours before vomiting will probably not have been absorbed. Report to prescriber. A replacement dose may be prescribed if an adverse drug reaction is not suspected. Severe vomiting and abdominal pain could represent pancreatitis or hepatitis.
Seizures worsening **Carbamazepine, tiagabine, gabapentin, vigabatrin or phenytoin can worsen absence or myoclonic seizures (also valproate in children)** **Ethosuximide can worsen generalised tonic-clonic seizures** **Lamotrigine co-administered with other antiepileptics can worsen seizure control**	Seizures should be monitored closely during initiation or change of therapy and puberty. Check temperature, particularly in children. Report urgently. Prescribers may request venous blood samples for liver function tests, particularly if valproate prescribed (below).
Seizures may occur more frequently during the premenstrual period and puberty	Ask patients to record medication use, seizures and menstruation in a diary or chart. Discuss problems with prescriber.

125

Rare adverse reactions: neuroleptic malignant syndrome, lung damage and joint pains reported with carbamazepine; neurological problems reported with valproate.

Box 14.2 Therapeutic monitoring

Measurement of the plasma concentration of antiepileptic drugs may be helpful:

◆ After dosage adjustments/initiation.
◆ In therapeutic failure/increased fits.
◆ During illness.
◆ To assess compliance.
◆ If signs of toxicity appear, including nystagmus, drowsiness, unsteadiness, double or blurred vision.
◆ If additional drugs are added or removed.
◆ In pregnancy and first 6 weeks after delivery.
◆ If disease present e.g. kidney or liver problems.
◆ Every 6 months with carbamazepine (NICE 2006b).

Cautions and contra-indications:

◆ **Previous adverse reactions** to the drug or related drug, e.g. carbamazepine is closely related to tricyclics, oxcarbazepine and phenytoin.

◆ **Liver/kidney impairment:** lower doses prescribed, choice of therapy will be restricted; measurements of plasma drug concentrations may be requested.

◆ **Pregnancy.** Specialist advice should be sought, preferably before conception. Medication requirements often change during pregnancy, and this requires monitoring by specialists. Folate supplements may be prescribed pre-conception to reduce the risk of neural tube defects (1% carbamazepine, 2–3% valproate) (Aronson 2006). Women should be advised that the fetus is more likely to be harmed by seizures than prescribed medication, and abrupt discontinuation of antiepileptics is hazardous. The risk of fetal malformations may be less with single-drug regimens (Morrell 2003). Mothers and neonates taking some antiepileptics (including carbamazepine, phenytoin) may be prescribed prophylactic vitamin K. Neonatal withdrawal problems (irritability, feeding problems, seizures) have occurred: delivery should be in specialist centres (Clerk & Emery 2002). Longterm follow up of infants may be advised.

◆ **Breastfeeding** of healthy infants may be possible with some antiepileptics. Infants must be carefully monitored for possible adverse effects, as problems can occur.

◆ **Children**: see manufacturers' guidelines.

◆ **Diabetes.** Urinalysis: valproate may cause false positives for ketones.

Gabapentin and phenytoin may affect control of diabetes.

◆ Further caveats are related to the adverse effect profiles of individual drugs, for example:

  ❖ **heart disease**, particularly heart block: carbamazepine
  ❖ **history of bone marrow suppression:** carbamazepine
  ❖ bleeding tendencies: valproate
  ❖ glaucoma: carbamazepine, topiramate
  ❖ neurological disorders: tiagabine
  ❖ history of psychosis: gabapentin
  ❖ porphyria (glossary): carbamazepine, oxcarbazepine, ethosuximide, phenytoin, valproate, some benzodiazepines
  ❖ thalassaemia: lamotrigine
  ❖ lupus: valproate
  ❖ congenital enzyme deficiencies, neurological disorders in children: valproate

126

Interactions (summary): Advise patients to inform prescribers and pharmacists of their anti-epileptic medication. Maintain detailed records on the effectiveness and adverse effects of both the anti-epileptic and the drug co-administered. Some drugs, including some antidepressants, antipsychotics, quinolones, antimalarials, amphetamines, high doses of caffeine, increase the risks of seizures. Anti-epileptic drugs interact with each other and special care is needed during addition or substitution of new drugs.

Alcohol may worsen drowsiness and incoordination, and intensify difficulties with driving.

Carbamazepine, phenytoin, topiramate, oxcarbazepine, barbiturates, and possibly lamotrigine, reduce the efficiency of **oral contraceptives** (including emergency hormonal contraceptives), necessitating higher doses. Advise women to seek advice should breakthrough bleeding occur (Fairgrieve *et al*. 2000). Women prescribed lamotrigine should discuss with prescribers before stopping the COC (dose of lamotrigine needs to be reduced).

Sedation, tremor and ataxia may be increased by benzodiazepines, other sedatives (see opioids), erythromycin, most SSRIs, clozapine, haloperidol, risperidone, paracetamol, omeprazole, amioradone, digoxin, nifedipine, and other drugs.

Bleeding and liver dysfunction due to valproate may be intensified by aspirin, salicylates, warfarin.

Grapefruit juice, influenza vaccine, caffeine may interact with carbamazepine.

Interactions may occur with folic acid, St. John's wort anti-cancer drugs, immunosuppressants, some corticosteroids, many anti-microbials e.g. aciclovir, metronidazole, doxycycline, azole antifungals

Contributor

Jeanette Hewitt RMN, RGN, RNT, BSc (Hons), PGCE, PGCertCouns. Lecturer, School of Health Sciences, Swansea University

15 Antibacterial drugs

Antibacterials are a diverse group of drugs which combat infections by suppressing the growth and reproduction of bacteria. However, many bacteria are now resistant to commonly used antibiotics (glossary) and some are resistant to all known agents. New drugs are continually being introduced to combat evolving patterns of resistance, mainly in gram-positive bacteria.

Actions: Antibiotics exploit the differences between bacterial and human cells. Some prevent the renewal of the bacterial cell wall (penicillins, cephalosporins, glycopeptides), while others inhibit protein formation within the bacteria (aminoglycosides, tetracyclines, macrolides).

Bacteria are 'gram negative' or 'gram positive'. Gram negative bacteria have a tough, complex wall, which can only be penetrated by the most powerful antibacterials, such as the aminoglycosides (e.g. gentamicin), quinolones. The tubercle *bacillus* is the most difficult of all to eradicate.

Indications (see Table 15.1):

Treating bacterial infections in accordance with culture and sensitivity testing or (second best) knowledge of prevalent organisms and distribution and activity of antibacterials. In severely ill patients, withholding therapy may result in failure to manage potentially serious or life-threatening infections, such as meningitis (Chambers 2006a). Broad spectrum antibiotics are used when the infectious agent is unknown. Narrow spectrum antibiotics are prescribed when the micro-organisms have been identified from tissue samples.

Prophylaxis:

◆ surgery e.g. gastrointestinal surgery, joint replacement.
◆ surgical/dental procedures in patients with artificial heart valvess or heart valve lesions.
◆ meningitis contacts

Administration:

◆ Dose depends on many factors: nature and severity of infection; weight (or ideal weight for height), age and renal function of patient. Some doses are determined by therapeutic monitoring undertaken on venous blood samples (e.g. gentamicin, teicoplanin, vancomycin). For aminoglycosides, these are extracted prior to dosing and one hour after dosing (BNF 2007).
◆ Crushing tablets or opening capsules allows growth of resistant micro-organisms on the skin or respiratory tract of the administrator.
◆ Gloves are worn when opening vials.

Table 15.1   Indications for some commonly prescribed antibacterials

Group and examples	Uses (examples only)
Beta lactams (penicillins, cephalosporins, carbapenems, monobactams)	Broad-spectrum antibiotics. Flucloxacillin and co-amoxiclav are effective against some penicillin-resistant organisms.
Aminoglycosides (gentamicin, amikacin, tobramycin)	Effective against gram negative bacteria e.g. *Pseudomonas sp.* Reserved for serious infections e.g. septicaemia, meningitis, hospital-acquired pneumonia.
Glycopeptides (vancomycin, teicoplanin)	Effective against staphylococci resistant to other drugs, including many strains of MRSA*. *Glycopeptides-resistant enterocicci are a major concern.*
Tetracyclines (doxycycline, minocycline)	Broad-spectrum antibiotics. Many indications, for example, genito-urinary infections, acne.
Macrolides (e.g. erythromycin)	Broad-spectrum antibiotics, prescribed for patients allergic to penicillin.
Metronidazole, tinidazole	Effective against anaerobic bacteria**. Prescribed for surgical prophylaxis, bacterial vaginosis, pressure sores, leg ulcers, dental abscess.
Quinolones (ciprofloxacin, ofloxacin)	Effective against gram negative bacteria, gonococci, gastrointestinal infections.
Streptogramins (quinupristin-dalfopristin)	Intravenous therapy for serious infections.
Lincosamides (clindamycin)	Serious infections. May be prescribed for resistant organisms or patients allergic to penicillins.
Linezolid and related drugs	Oral or intravenous therapy for serious infections resistant to other agents.
Antitubercular drugs (rifampicin, isoniazid, rifabutin, streptomycin)	Reserved for treatment/containment of tuberculosis (TB).
Sulphonamides (co-trimoxazole)	Reserved for serious infections associated with HIV/AIDS.
Trimethoprin	Urinary tract infections.
Chloramphenicol	Mainly used for eye infections.

* Many bacteria produce an enzyme which destroys beta lactam antibiotics. In addition to this, MRSA (meticillin-resistant *Staphylococcus aureus)* produces an inactivating protein which confers resistance to most other antibiotics.
** Anaerobic bacteria grow in oxygen-poor environments, such as the gut or wounds. Examples include *Clostridia sp., Bacteroides sp.*

♦ Severe infections require intravenous infusion. Observe veins carefully for signs of phlebitis, particularly with prolonged administration, penicillins or vancomycin.

♦ Intramuscular injections are painful and avoided, where possible, in children. A warm compress may reduce pain (Smith *et al.* 2008). (Figure 21.1)

♦ Food affects absorption of orally administered drugs (see Table 15.2).

Table 15.2 Oral administration

Drug	Potential Problem	Precaution
Tetracyclines Quinolones	Absorption impaired by iron, zinc or calcium in the stomach	Taken either 1 hour before or 2 hours after tablets containing minerals or dairy products
Doxycycline Minocycline	Oesophageal or gastric irritation	Swallowed whole, taken with food and a full glass of water (Box 1.1)
Ampicillin Macrolides (some forms of erythromycin) Rifampicin	Absorption reduced by food in the stomach	Taken 1 hour before or 2 hours after meals
Amoxycillin	Absorption reduced by high fibre diets, e.g. bran or bulk laxatives e.g. methylcellulose	Dose increases may be required
Most antibacterials and azole antifungals	Absorption impaired by antacids, particularly those containing magnesium and aluminium	Antibiotic taken 2–3 hours apart from antacids

(Schmidt & Dalhoff 2002, Chambers 2006b)

130

Adverse effects:

Adverse effects of antibiotics can be considered as:

♦ those occurring with all antibiotics.

♦ those restricted to specific drugs, which may accumulate in certain tissues or directly damage certain cells.

Superinfection is a new infection emerging during therapy of a primary infection. The normal micro-organisms are removed, allowing others to invade, such as fungi (e.g. *Candida sp.*– thrush), *Pseudomonas sp.*, *Chlostridium sp.* or Enterobacteria. The new micro-organisms are likely to be drug-resistant.

Adverse effects: implications for practice: ANTIBACTERIALS

Most, but not all, of these are more likely with high doses and prolonged use.

Potential Problem	Suggestions for Prevention and Management
Problems associated with all antibacterials	
Superinfection	
Diarrhoea/gastrointestinal upset **This may be dose-related, due to direct action on the gut wall (beta lactams, clindamycin) or due to overgrowth of pathogenic micro-organisms (at any dose). Problems may occur with all routes of administration**	Minimise use of broad-spectrum antibiotics. Monitor fluid and electrolyte balance if diarrhoea and vomiting occur and be alert for *Chlostridium difficile* infections. These may not respond to initial therapy. Probiotic supplements may help to prevent antibiotic associated diarrhoea (Sazawal *et al.* 2006). Certain bacterial strains were effective when taken in the first 48 hours of antibiotic therapy until 1 week after discontinuation (Hickson *et al.* 2007). Small frequent meals may alleviate gastrointestinal disturbance.
Fungal infections e.g. stomatitis from oral thrush	Offer ice cubes. Maintain mouth care.
Reactivation of dormant infections	If aminoglycosides are administered, monitor for worsening of TB and *Herpes* infections.
Therapeutic failure	
Infection persists	Check: ◆ drug, dose, route. Drug administered may not be reaching the micro-organism e.g. intracellular organisms such as salmonella, TB, listeria ◆ drug resistance/tolerance ◆ superinfection – repeat swab ◆ undetected micro-organisms – repeat swab ◆ administration problems e.g. incompatibilities, interactions ◆ foreign body e.g. prostheses, catheters (Pratt *et al.* 2007) ◆ pus or haematoma or abscess formation prevents drugs from reaching micro-organisms; doctors may decide that surgical drainage is necessary. Discuss, with prescribers, the possibility of compromise of the immune system. Venous blood samples may be required.
Certain antibacterials, particularly aminoglycosides, have a narrow margin between therapeutic dose and toxicity	Check: ◆ inadequate dosage or compliance/ administration ◆ Dosage schedule – drug concentration falling below the minimum effective concentration
Meningitis As inflammation subsides, the blood/brain barrier	Monitor closely for signs of relapse. Ensure therapy continues until patient is well.

becomes less permeable. The drugs may then fail to reach their target	
Resistance **The relevant genetic information can spread rapidly between different micro-organisms**	Minimise antibiotic use unless bacterial sensitivity is known. Ensure adequate doses, making allowances for drug-food interactions. Complete the course. Observe hospital policies for hand-washing, asepsis, and single-use equipment. Scrupulous care of indwelling catheters (Pratt *et al.* 2007). Biofilms impenetrable to antibacterials form on the surfaces. Try to prevent contact between MRSA and vancomycin-resistant enterococci by separating patients harbouring these bacteria. Such contact could allow development of vancomycin-resistant MRSA.
Hypersensitivity (chapter 21)	
Rash, angioedema, anaphylaxis, or other signs and symptoms, see Table 21.1. 1–4% of courses of penicillins are complicated by allergic reactions (Petri 2006)	Thorough patient history. Pre-therapy assessment of breathing pattern and skin to facilitate detection of any changes. Check all skin, particularly pressure areas, for emergence of rashes. Administer intravenous therapy slowly. Advise patients that rashes may persist for weeks after discontinuation. Skin tests are available to predict allergy to penicillins, but not other drugs.
Drug fever	Discuss, with prescriber, the possibility of a hypersensitivity response, and, consequently, the need to discontinue administration. Be aware that this could be confused with renewed infection (Chambers 2006a).

132

Problems associated with specific antibacterials		
Potential problem/ damage	**Drug**	**Suggestions for Prevention and Management**
Convulsions	Penicillins Cephalosporins other betalactams Quinolones	Caution in patients with histories of convulsions and/or renal failure. Cautious co-administration of quinolones and NSAIDs, particularly fenbufen, or theophylline.
Confusion, delirium	Aminoglycosides Macrolides	Check renal function and drug interactions.

Peripheral nerves, causing pain, numbness, tingling	Aminoglycosides, linezolid, isoniazid, metronidazole (rare)	Ask patient to report any abnormal sensation in fingers or feet. Alternative drugs may be needed. Isoniazid may be administered with pyridoxine, vitamin B$_6$.
Optic nerve	Linezolid Antitubercular drugs	Enquire regarding any changes or blurring of vision and report urgently. After 28 days' therapy, arrange for monitoring of vision (BNF 2007).
Inner ear Hearing loss initially affects high tones, but may spread to frequencies used in speech. Loss of balance, preceded by headache and emesis. Recovery of sense of balance may take months or be incomplete.	Gentamicin and other aminoglycosides Vancomycin Rarely: Erythromycin Minocycline	Avoid co-administration of other drugs affecting the ear (interactions). Avoid in pregnancy and breastfeeding, if possible. Administer intravenous therapy slowly. Ensure patient can hear and balance is not affected. Mobilise carefully. Inquire about tinnitus. Report to prescriber. If drug is not discontinued promptly, hearing loss may be irreversible. Aminoglycosides: ◆ Report any headache to prescriber. ◆ Duration of therapy should be minimised.
Tendons	Quinolones	Usually avoided in children & those prescribed corticosteroids. Pain & soreness over Achilles' tendon should be reported immediately.
Cardiac dysrhythmia	Clindamycin, some quinolones, erythromycin (rarely)	Administer intravenous preparations slowly.
Liver	Erythromycin Rifampicin Isoniazid Rarely: Tetracyclines Cephalosporins Co-amoxiclav	Be prepared to undertake liver function tests if use prolonged. Obtain history of alcohol use. Prescriber may select alternative therapy for heavy users.
Pancreas	Co-trimoxazole	Be alert for severe vomiting and acute abdominal pain radiating to the back. Arrange venous blood samples for glucose and amylase estimation.

Kidney	Gentamicin Vancomycin Co-trimoxazole Rarely: Cephalosporins Penicillins Tetracyclines Quinolones	Check serum creatinine and urea to assess renal function before and during therapy (chapter 21). Prescribers may select alternative drug for older adults. Ensure adequate hydration, including replacing any losses due to diarrhoea and vomiting.
Dark urine	Metronidazole	Advise patients using long-term metronidazole that this is a harmless reaction.
Loss of magnesium	Gentamicin, long-term administration to older people	Be prepared to organise venous blood samples and urine collection for laboratory assessment of magnesium concentrations.
Bleeding Both platelets and clotting factors may be affected	Beta lactams Linezolid Vancomycin	Check platelets. Check skin for purpura. In acute settings, clotting factor concentrations may be measured. Particular care if patients are taking anticoagulants (Petri 2006).
Skin (photosensitivity)	Tetracyclines, Quinolones, Clindamycin	Advise covering skin with clothing and high factor, high star sunscreen during exposure to direct sunlight. Warn patients of possible discolouration with long-term minocycline.
Bone marrow: Platelets White cells (neutrophils)	Chloramphenicol Co-trimoxazole Linezolid Rarely: Cephalosporins Aminoglycosides Vancomycin	Patients with history/family history of blood dyscrasias or taking other drugs potentially toxic to the bone marrow (e.g. carbimazole, carbamazepine, antipsychotics) may be prescribed alternative agents. Check FBC routinely and if sore throat or fever develop. Linezolid: pre-therapy and weekly full blood counts (BNF 2007).

Cautions and contra-indications:

◆ **History of hypersensitivity.** Patients allergic to cephalosporins are often allergic to penicillins and *vice versa*. Patients allergic to diuretics, celecoxib or oral hypogly-caemics may be allergic to sulphonamides.

◆ **Glandular fever** (Epstein-Barr virus infection), **cytomegalovirus** infection, HIV or chronic lymphatic leukaemia greatly increase the risk of developing a penicillin-induced rash, particularly ampicillin.

- **Impaired renal function** causes some drugs to accumulate e.g. penicillins, tetracyclines, vancomycin, ciprofloxacin, teicoplanin. Injectable penicillins contain sodium, which may contribute to fluid retention.
- **Impaired liver function** causes some drugs to accumulate e.g. metronidazole, rifampicin.
- **Myasthenia gravis.** Aminoglycosides and quinolones exacerbate this condition.
- **Porphyria** (glossary). Avoid sulphonamides, cephalosporins, erythromycin, flucloxacillin, rifampicin, trimethoprin.
- **Pregnancy:** Penicillins are usually the antibiotics of first choice. Tetracyclines, trimethoprin, co-trimazole, glycopeptides and aminoglycosides are avoided if possible. See table pp. 306–7 in Jordan (2002b).
- **Breastfeeding** allows small amounts of antibacterial to pass from mother to infant. Hypersensitivity responses and adverse effects may occur in the infant. Breastfeeding is not advised in some severe infections.
- **Penicillins** are not given by the intrathecal route, due to the risk of convulsions.

Interactions (summary): Antibacterials interact with a wide variety of other drugs and chemicals including alcohol, nutrients, oral contraceptives, anticoagulants, digoxin, lithium and many drugs administered in intensive care (Pea & Furlanut 2001).

- Adverse effects are cumulative when drugs causing similar problems are co-administered. For example, drugs damaging the inner ear (e.g. gentamicin, vancomycin, teicoplanin, cisplatin, furosemide), are rarely combined. Similarly, co-administration of drugs damaging the kidney is avoided, if possible, for example, gentamicin, cisplatin, furosemide, daunorubicin, NSAIDs.
- Susceptible people suffer an 'antabuse-like reaction' if they take even a small amount of alcohol with certain anti-microbials, usually metronidazole, but also tinidazole, ketoconazole (an antifungal). This results in dilatation of all the blood vessels, causing flushing, severe headache and profound hypotension. Faints, falls and cardiovascular collapse may follow (Baxter 2006).
- Oral contraceptives.
  - ❖ Rifampicin and rifabutin render all oral contraceptives ineffective.
  - ❖ All broad-spectrum antibiotics increase the risk of 'pill failure' for combined oral contraceptives. Additional contraception recommended during and up to 7 days after course of antibacterials completed. If the 7 days is beyond the end of the packet, avoid a break between packets (BNF 2007).
- Many antibacterials are incompatible with other drugs when co-administered in intravenous infusions. For example, if gentamicin is combined with heparin or a penicillin, its activity will be lost.
- **Surgery.** Aminoglycosides and vancomycin intensify the action of muscle relaxants such as suxamethonium. All muscle relaxants interact with clindomycin, piperacillin, polymixins. Highlight use when transferring patients to anaesthetic teams.
- Macrolides cause accumulation of other drugs e.g. digoxin, corticosteroids, anticoagulants, ciclosporin, SSRIs, some statins. Metronidazole interacts similarly with carbamazepine, ciclosporin, lithium, tacrolimus.

- ◆ Cardiac dysrhythmias are more likely if quinolones are co-administered with several drugs e.g. antipsychotics, amiodarone, some antidepressants.
- ◆ Betalactams and metronidazole may enhance or inhibit anticoagulants.
- ◆ Linezolid is an MAOI (monoamino oxidase inhibitor). Ingestion of preparations containing tyramine may cause severe hypertension. Patients should avoid tyramine-rich foods, such as marmite, mature cheese, alcohol (except spirits), 'cold cures', cocaine, amphetamines. Problems may arise with co-administration of pethidine, antidepressants, triptans, levo-dopa, salbutamol.

The care of patients with TB, severe viral and fungal infections is undertaken in specialist units. Specialist literature should be consulted.

Contributor

John Knight BSc, PhD. Lecturer, School of Health Sciences, Swansea University

16 Insulin

Insulin is prescribed to compensate for the total or partial failure of the pancreas that occurs in diabetes mellitus.

Diabetes is diagnosed in symptomatic individuals if:

◆ fasting (>8 hours since intaking calories) venous plasma glucose >7.0 mmol/l

◆ or random (any time) venous plasma glucose is >11.1 mmol/l.

◆ or whole blood glucose >6.1 and 10.0 mmol/l.

◆ or capillary whole blood glucose >6.1 and >11.1 mmol/l.

Lower fasting plasma glucose concentrations, possibly as low as 5.05–5.50 mmol/l, indicate impaired glucose tolerance, and the need for further monitoring (Frier & Fisher 2002, Genuth et al. 2003).

Actions: Insulin is the 'storage' hormone, normally secreted after meals. It alters the directions of the metabolic pathways, so that sugars, fats and amino acids are removed from the circulation, transported into cells for storage, and not used as sources of energy. This allows the body to:

◆ form fat stores, and gain weight.

◆ use amino acids for growth or healing.

◆ remove glucose from the circulation and tissues.

◆ move potassium ions into the cells.

Without insulin, the cells starve, while blood glucose, cholesterol and triglyceride (fats) concentrations increase.

After a meal, blood glucose concentration rises. Insulin returns it to normal within 2 hours. In health, about 50% of the body's insulin (totalling 18–40 units/day) is secreted at a basal rate of 0.5–1 unit/hour, and the remainder is secreted in response to meals at 5–6 units/hour. It is not always possible to achieve this pattern by insulin injections.

Insulin is secreted by the pancreas into the hepatic portal vein. Therefore, it passes directly to the liver, where it exerts its effects and is destroyed, before reaching the general circulation. This direct effect is not achieved when insulin is injected into skin or veins. This partly explains why people who inject insulin do not regulate their blood sugar concentrations as closely or as well as people with a healthy pancreas, and, consequently, suffer higher rates of cardiovascular disease.

Indications and administration: Diabetes:

◆ Type 1. All insulin-producing cells are destroyed. Manufactured insulin is needed from the time of diagnosis.

◆ Type 2. Insufficient insulin is produced and cells fail to respond to insulin. Manufactured insulin is often needed, particularly during illness.

◆ Other types, for example, destruction of the pancreas by cystic fibrosis, cancer or pancreatitis. Insulin replacement therapy is required.

Blood glucose concentrations should be monitored and maintained between 4–8 mmol/l before meals and below 10 mmol/l after meals in children and 4–7 mmol/l before meals and below 9 mmol/l after meals in adults (NICE 2004d).

Insulin is usually injected subcutaneously into the thigh, abdominal wall, gluteal or deltoid regions. Sites are rotated, and selected consistently according to time of day (Figure 16.1):

◆ Insulin is absorbed most rapidly from the abdomen, the usual site for the first morning injection and mealtime injections in adults.

◆ Exercise increases insulin absorption from the limbs, and these sites are best avoided before exercise. The final injection of the day is often into the thigh (Davis 2006).

> Sites for subcutaneous administration.
>
> By numbering the areas, it is possible to ensure that injections are rotated within each area, and not administered on the site of a recent injection. This is important if injections are administered long-term, particularly for insulin therapy. Injection sites should be 1 inch (2.4 centimetres) apart.

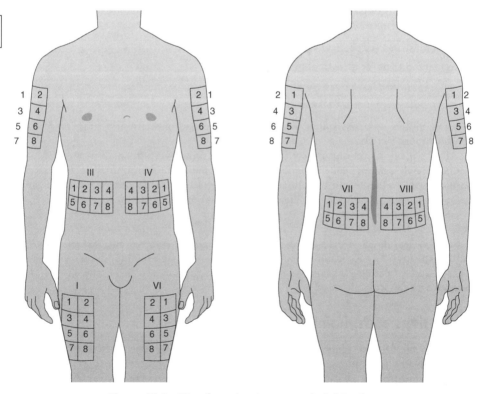

Figure 16.1   Sites for subcutaneous administration

A wide variety of insulin preparations is available.

◆ Preparations should be checked with patients, carers and colleagues before administration.

◆ Insulin is often injected into lifted skin folds, to minimise unintended intra-muscular administration.

◆ Needle length is selected in accordance with depth of subcutaneous fat (NICE 2004d) (Figure 10.4).

◆ The needle is held in place for 6–10 seconds, or 10–30 seconds with some pens, to ensure the entire dose is injected.

◆ After injecting, pressure is applied for several seconds, without rubbing.

Some patients prefer the more convenient 'insulin pens' to traditional syringes: pens may improve compliance, but not disease control (Korytkowski et al. 2003).

Speed of action depends on type of insulin (Table 16.1).

Table 16.1 Properties of insulin preparations (some examples)

Insulin type	Onset (minutes)	Peak (hours)	Duration (hours)	Time of injection
Fast acting				
Aspart	5–15	0.5–0.66* 0.8–1.5**	4–6	Immediately before or soon after meals
Lispro	5–15	0.5–1.17*	3–5	Immediately before or soon after meals
Short acting				
Soluble	30–45	1.5–4	5–8	30–45 minutes before meals
Intermediate				
Isophane (NPH)	60–120	6–12	12–18	Set times of day
Insulin zinc suspension (Lente)	60–120	6–12	12–20	Set times of day
Long acting				
Insulin glargine	70	5–24 hours, no peak	20–24+	Once daily, same time

* type 1 diabetes
** type 2 diabetes

Figures from manufacturers' data sheets (ABPI 2007), Hirsch (2005) and Davis (2006 p.1625)

Insulin lispro and aspart act more rapidly and briefly than soluble insulin. This is useful for people who do not plan their meals or wish to eat late at night. If food intake cannot be predicted, these insulins can be given after food, with a dose based on actual, rather than predicted, intake. This is helpful to young children (NICE 2004d) or those with poor appetite secondary to autonomic nervous system dysfunction caused by diabetes.

Most patients receive both short- or fast-acting insulin plus intermediate insulin. Certain combinations can be mixed before administration, according to manufacturers' instructions. Insulin mixtures: intermediate and long-acting insulins should be mixed thoroughly until uniformly cloudy by rotating and gently inverting the insulin container 20 times (Jehle *et al.* 1999). Shaking causes foaming: bubbles prevent administration of accurate doses.

Type and dose are determined by specialists, according to: weight, age, growth, fitness, diet, lifestyle, other medications, any insulin antibodies, treatment response. Total requirements usually range 0.5–1.0 international units/kg/day, 0.7–1.0 international units/kg/day for pre-pubertal children and up to 2 units/kg/day for obese patients. Insulin pens deliver 1–60 units.

Absorption of insulin varies with:

◆ Injection: dose, depth, site, volume. If injected into muscle, long-acting insulin may be absorbed twice as rapidly as when injected subcutaneously.

◆ Individual: age (slower in older people), condition (slower in type 2), amount of subcutaneous fat, insulin antibodies.

◆ Blood supply: skin temperature, physical activity, massage, vasodilatation (for example, alcohol, pregnancy), vasoconstriction (for example, nicotine, shock), position (standing reduces blood flow to legs and abdomen). Smoking contracts blood vessels and decreases absorption of insulin.

Soluble insulin is administered intravenously to manage acute hyperglycaemia and keto-acidosis or during surgery, illness or labour. It acts almost immediately and lasts about 30 minutes.

Portable infusion pumps deliver continuous basal infusions of short-acting insulin with patient-activated boluses at mealtimes. Specialists prescribe these to overcome recurrent, unpredictable hypoglycaemia in patients able to monitor blood glucose closely (NICE 2004d). Alternative insulin and clear protocols to prevent severe hyperglycaemia must be available, should the pump fail, the line block or leak, or the needle become dislodged. Careful handling is needed to avoid abscess formation or local infection. Introduction of the incorrect insulin can block the tubing. Seek specialist advice before using at high altitude.

Inhaled insulin was formerly prescribed by specialists for certain adults (NICE 2006c). At the time of writing, it is not avalaible in the UK.

Storage should be at 2–8°C, without freezing. Once opened, most insulins should be stored below 30°C (<25°C for insulin glargine) outside the refrigerator, protected from light, and used within 28 days. Some manufacturers recommend keeping insulin at room temperature for 1–2 hours before injection. Inhaled insulin should not be refrigerated or exposed to moisture.

Adverse effects:

◆ **Hypoglycaemia.** Insulin transfers glucose from the blood into the cells. If the insulin dose is too high, the concentration of glucose in the blood falls too low, and the brain will have insufficient energy to function normally. The glucose concentration at which a hypoglycaemic response occurs depends on the individual; it is normally around 2.6 mmol/l, but may be higher in people with diabetes. In health, between meals, a fall in blood glucose concentration triggers secretion of the hormone glucagon. This stimulates the liver to release more glucose from glycogen stores, into the circulation to prevent hypoglycaemia. This response becomes deficient in people with type 1 diabetes, and adrenaline is secreted to correct hypoglycaemia. Adrenaline is the hormone of fright or flight (see broncho-dilators), and causes many of the symptoms associated with hypoglycaemia, such as sweating, palor, palpitations, anxiety, shaking. With repeated hypoglycaemia, release of adrenaline may become deficient, the patient loses hypoglycaemia awareness, and is vulnerable to severe episodes, without warning.

◆ Insulin can cause weight gain and acts on the kidneys to inhibit excretion of salt and water, which can cause oedema.

Adverse effects: implications for practice:

Potential Problem	Suggestions for Prevention and Management
Hypoglycaemia	
Warning signs and symptoms: anxiety, fatigue, blurred or double vision, cold sweats, palor, confusion, nausea, difficulty concentrating, accidents, aggression, drowsiness, headache, tachycardia, palpitations, shaking, weakness, mental impairment, yawning, speech difficulties, numbness of fingers. **Within hours, untreated hypoglycaemia causes loss of consciousness, convulsions and, if prolonged, neurological damage, particularly in individuals with pre-existing vascular disease or children under 7.**	Ensure patients are aware of: ◆ warning signs and symptoms ◆ the need to have carbohydrates available at all times e.g. sugar lumps. ◆ protocols (BNF 2007) **Risk factors:** ◆ Injections: excessive doses, inadequately mixed suspensions, changes in administration, brand, source or type of insulin. ◆ Behaviour: excessive exercise (often several hours earlier or within 1–3 hours of lispro or aspart administration), anorexia, omitting food, particularly supper, drinking alcohol. ◆ Illness: vomiting, patients with type 2 diabetics starting insulin (overnight administration may help), malnutrition, recovery from infection, surgery or termination of pregnancy. Discuss, with prescriber, need to test for pregnancy, liver disease, kidney disease, hypothyroidism, other endocrine conditions. Advise patients to record the time of day of all episodes in a diary, so that any relationship to time of injection may be ascertained. Report mild hypoglycaemia, because this often precedes serious episodes (Aronson 2006). Advise 'medi-alert' identification.
Accidents, impaired reaction times	Driving is restricted (BNF 2007). Glucose concentrations should be checked before driving and every 2 hours. Supplies of glucose should always be available.
Hearing loss, temporary	Patients need to be aware of this threat to safety during periods of hypoglycaemia (Strachan *et al.* 2003).
Cardiac event, such as heart attack or angina	Warn patients that these problems may be caused by hypoglycaemia.

Hypoglycaemic episode **If the patient does not respond to treatment, the prescriber may consider alternative explanations, such as a cardiovascular event**	Summon appropriate medical assistance. Conscious patients should ingest **carbohydrates**, such as 3–6 sugar lumps, or glucose-rich liquids. Additional carbohydrate should be eaten e.g. 200–400ml milk, sandwiches. Recheck glucose concentrations within 10–15 minutes. If the gag reflex is doubtful, glucose gels can be applied to the gums. In semi-conscious/unconscious patients, glucagon may be injected, followed by intravenous glucose, if no response within 10–15 minutes. **Glucagon** may not be effective in patients who have ingested alcohol, not eaten and those with type 2 diabetes. It may cause emesis. Hypoglycaemia may recur several hours after apparent recovery; therefore observations should be maintained (BNF 2007).
Nocturnal hypoglycaemia (highest risk 4–7.30 a.m.) **Symptoms:** ◆ **nightmares,** ◆ **night sweats (or wet bedclothes),** ◆ **morning headache, tiredness.**	Ensure prescriber is informed of any symptoms. Ask patient to check blood glucose on waking in the night or just before retiring. Ensure supper is provided, particularly for those using regular insulin at evening meal (Hirsch 2005). Advise against alcohol ingestion. Discuss, with prescriber, substitution of fast-acting insulin (aspart or lispro) at evening meal and the prescription of insulin glargine (NICE 2004d, Davis 2006).
Behaviour disturbance/ aggression/psychosis	Document in diary to facilitate recognition of links to hypoglycaemia. Monitor blood glucose closely over 24 hours.
Insulin overdose, either accidental or associated with attempted suicide	To reduce potential errors, establish a routine and keep to same brands of insulin, syringes, needles and order of administration. Check these with patients before administration.
Loss of hypoglycaemia awareness/warning, associated with: repeated episodes, age, damage to the autonomic nervous system caused by long-standing diabetes	Inform patient that driving is prohibited (BNF 2007). Review any intensified insulin therapy or change of insulin. Encourage patients to avoid any hypoglycaemia for 3 months, in an attempt to improve awareness (Aronson 2006).
Change in body fat and fluids	
Weight gain (DCCTRG 2001), leading to: **worsening diabetes; risk of cardiovascular disease**	Monitor weight and girth closely (see oral anti-diabetic agents). Extra care if insulin is introduced alongside sulphonylureas.
Alteration in body image	Be aware that adolescents may withhold their insulin to lose weight.

Peripheral oedema and vision difficulties	Report to physician: dose of insulin may be excessive. May subside within days of initiation of therapy.
Postural hypotension, in long-standing diabetes, exacerbated by insulin	Check BP lying and standing. Advise clients to rise slowly. Extra care if anti-hypertensives, antipsychotics or antidepressants are co-prescribed.

Injection sites

Lipodystrophy (subcutaneous lumps)	Prevention: rotate injections within each site (Figure 16.1). Separate injections by 2.5cm (1 inch). Do not reuse site for 1 month. Avoid injecting into lumps.
Subcutaneous fat deposition (lipohypertrophy), due to local action of insulin	Prevention: rotate sites. Avoid injecting into hypertrophied sites, as absorption is delayed.
Lipoatrophy (rare) or atrophy of subcutaneous fat may be due to insulin antibodies	Seek specialist advice. Siting of injections may allow restoration of fat (Davis 2006).
Bruising, redness, pain, swelling, itching Problems may be due to allergy and may be transient	Check sites regularly. Re-assess injection and skin cleansing techniques. Clean skin with non-irritant solution. Ensure injection is not too superficial. Antihistamine or hydrocortisone creams may reduce discomfort. Discuss, with prescriber, the possibility that the problem is due to an excipient, such as zinc or protamine.

Insulin infusions

Hypokalaemia (glossary) as potassium is transferred into cells	Ensure serum potassium is closely monitored and potassium is replaced accordingly.
Insulin may adhere to plastic giving sets	Titrate infusions to patient's response and blood glucose concentration. Insulin is not added directly to fluid bags (NICE 2004d).
Hypoglycaemia Behaviour disturbance/ aggression due to excess insulin causing hypoglycaemia	Ensure glucose concentrations are closely monitored and dextrose infusions are administered as prescribed.
Relapse after discontinuation of infusion	Ensure any prescribed subcutaneous insulin is administered at least 30 minutes before infusion is discontinued (Davis 2006).

Therapeutic failure	
Hyperglycaemia. If not actioned, ketoacidosis within days	Monitor patients closely during acute illness, infection, emotional stress, trauma, surgery, heart attack and puberty.
	Ensure that patients respond to the earliest signs of infection, and note these in their diary.
	Advise patients of the warning signs: drowsiness, 'not coping', anorexia, nausea, abdominal pain, increased urination and thirst.
	Discuss, with prescriber, the possibility of insulin resistance, and the need for increased doses.
	Consider the possibility of eating disorders or deliberate withholding of insulin to control body weight.
Pre-breakfast hyperglycaemia. This is due to the natural 24 hour endocrine rhythm	Discuss with prescriber use of insulin glargine (NICE 2004d). This may be associated with potentially dangerous nocturnal hypoglycaemia, above.
Poor control of diabetes and long-term complications (UKPDS Group 1998)	Monitor the progress of the disease regularly, including assessment of cardiovascular system, kidneys, eyes, dental health, growth, thyroid function, coeliac disease (NICE 2004d).
Varying therapeutic response, due to changes in absorption (up to 50% in any individual)	Plan regular patterns of eating, exercise, sleep and injections.

Generalised hypersensitivity responses to insulin are rare (<1 in 10,000). Other rare adverse effects include liver damage, muscle breakdown.

Cautions and contra-indications:

◆ **Previous hypersensitivity** responses to insulin or other components of injections.

◆ **Pregnant and breastfeeding** women receive specialist care. Intensive monitoring is essential to avoid hypoglycaemia in the first trimester and hyperglycaemia in the second and third trimesters (Jordan 2002b).

◆ **Children.** Doses are adjusted by specialists, in relation to growth, development and puberty. Some preparations are not recommended by manufacturers.

◆ **Kidney or liver (usually) impairment, coeliac disease or Addison's disease** reduce insulin requirements.

◆ Gastrointestinal disorders causing delayed absorption of food may restrict the use of fast-acting insulins.

◆ Patients with Raynaud's phenomenon may find that blood glucose monitoring gives inaccurate results (too low). Rubbing the arm may help. Specialists may advise automated sensor systems.

◆ **Inhaled insulin** was contra-indicated in patients with severe respiratory conditions, smokers, and those who had smoked within the last 6 months. Absorption was increased by smoking and decreased by exposure to tobacco smoke. Manufacturers recommended pre-therapy and follow-up lung function tests (ABPI, Exubera®, 2007).

Interactions (summary): Monitor blood glucose closely to detect any:

- **Hyperglycaemia** associated with: thiazides, thyroid hormones, amphetamines, cocaine, salbutamol, large quantities of caffeine, growth hormone, oestrogens, chlorpromazine, clozapine, olanzapine, lithium, corticosteroids, calcium channel antagonists, danazol, marijuana, nicotine, medicines containing sugar.
- **Hypoglycaemia** associated with: ACE inhibitors, salicylates (effects minimal), anabolic steroids, monoamine oxidise inhibitors, lithium, octreotide, disopyramide, cyclophosphamide, pentamidine, pyridoxine, tetracyclines (rare). Bronchodilators increase absorption of inhaled insulin.
- **Excess alcohol consumption** prolongs and/or delays hypoglycaemia. Alcohol should be taken with food and limited to 2–3 drinks/day. Avoid driving (Baxter 2006).
- **Beta blockers** and clonidine may: mask warnings of hypoglycaemia; delay recovery from hypoglycaemia; cause hypertension during hypoglycaemia. Selective beta blockers, such as atenolol, cause fewer problems.

145

Contributor

Richard Lake RN, Dip.N, BSc (Hons), ATNC Clinical Skills Tutor, School of Health Sciences, Swansea University

17 Oral Anti-diabetic drugs

Oral anti-diabetic drugs may be prescribed for people with type 2 diabetes. They increase the response to any remaining insulin and/or stimulate the pancreatic output of insulin. (See Table 17.1.)

Oral medication is usually prescribed in conjunction with exercise and diet regimens (Oiknine & Mooradian 2003). Therapy may be short- or long-term. If type 2 diabetes progresses, the pancreas becomes exhausted, and insulin is needed. For every 6 years of type 2 diabetes, the ability of the pancreas to secrete insulin declines by 50% (Davis 2006).

Indications and administration: Anti-diabetic drugs may be prescribed alone or, if monotherapy is ineffective, in combinations, in accordance with current guidelines. They include:

♦ **Sulphonylureas**, e.g. glibenclamide, glimepiride, gliclazide, glipizide, tolbutamide, gliquidone, chlorpropamide (no longer recommended): prescribed if metformin unsuitable, for example, patients with mild renal impairment. Administered with breakfast and other meals, if necessary. Gliquidone and glipizide are taken before meals. Food may reduce absorption.

♦ **Metformin:** first choice for overweight patients (NICE 2002). Administered with food.

♦ **Acarbose:** often combined with other drugs, but may be first drug prescribed. Chewed with first mouthful of food or swallowed with liquid just before meals.

♦ **Meglitinides** e.g. repaglinide, nateglinide: sometimes prescribed in combination with metformin. Administered 1–30 minutes before main meals.

♦ **Thiazolidinediones**, e.g. pioglitazone: prescribed under limited circumstances for patients unable to tolerate metformin or sulphonylureas. Administration not restricted.

Table 17.1 Oral anti-diabetic agents compared

Drug	Main Action	Weight increase	Main problems
Sulphonylureas	Stimulate insulin release, decrease insulin breakdown	Yes	Risk of prolonged hypoglycaemia with excessive doses.
Metformin	Decreases glucose formation in the liver. Enhances insulin's actions in fat and muscle.	No	Risk of lactic acidosis (rare) if patient becomes unwell, intakes excess alcohol or develops renal impairment.
Acarbose	Inhibits digestion of carbohydrate	No	Flatulence, diarrhoea. Effects on blood glucose concentrations modest.

Meglitinides	Stimulate insulin release	Yes	Hypoglycaemia, hypersensitivity.
Thiazolidinediones	Augment insulin's actions in tissues.	Yes	Diabetes may worsen. Oedema/worsening of heart failure. Hypoglycaemia.

(Oiknine & Mooradian 2003, Davis 2006)

Adverse effects:

◆ **Hypoglycaemia** can occur with sulphonylureas, thiazolidinediones, meglitinides, combination therapies.

◆ **Cardiovascular disease.** Maintaining blood glucose concentrations within normal limits is important in the prevention of cardiovascular, kidney and eye disease and for the immune system and healing. However, oral anti-diabetic agents may adversely affect some risk factors, such as weight and lipid profile, without being fully effective in reducing glucose concentrations. Drugs which stimulate or mimic the actions of insulin will inevitably increase fat stores and stimulate hunger (and eating). A large study found no difference in mortality between treatments (UKPDS 1998).

◆ **Gastrointestinal tract.** Most agents can cause gastrointestinal upset.

◆ Some sulphonylureas may stimulate secretion of ADH (see SIADH, anti-depressants).

Metformin inhibits liver enzymes, including those which metabolise lactic acid, and can, rarely, allow this to accumulate, causing '**lactic acidosis**'. This restricts the use of metformin, see cautions.

Adverse effects: implications for practice

Potential Problem	Suggestions for Prevention and Management
Hypoglycaemia (see insulin)	
Warning signs and symptoms: **anxiety, fatigue, nightmares, accidents, blurred vision, cold sweats, pallor, confusion, difficulty concentrating, headache, tachycardia, shaking, weakness, mental impairment**	Ensure patients are aware of warning signs and symptoms. Advise against: ◆ exceeding prescribed dose, even if a previous dose has been forgotten. ◆ omitting meals. ◆ taking alcohol without food. ◆ severe, prolonged exercise. Do not administer meglitinides or acarbose if meals are missed or vomited.

May progress to:	Advise patients to:
Impaired reactions, collapse, coma and neurological damage Estimated to occur in 0.3% patients prescribed sulphonylureas in first 8 weeks of therapy (Aronson 2006)	◆ balance energy intake throughout the day ◆ ensure supplies of glucose are always available, particularly if driving ◆ wear 'medi-alert' identification.
Hypoglycaemic episode **Hypoglycaemia may be prolonged or return**	Seek urgent medical advice. Administer oral glucose, if appropriate. Sucrose e.g. sugar, will be indigestible and ineffective if acarbose has been taken. Intravenous glucose may be needed. Avoid glucagon (BNF 2007). Following initial treatment, transfer to hospital is advised.
Vision disturbance	Advise patients this may be caused by changes in blood glucose, and may resolve. Check blood glucose.
Neurological disturbance, such as headache, fatigue, tremor, signs and symptoms of a stroke **Paraesthesia with thiazolidinediones and sulphonylureas** **Drowsiness with glipizide**	Check blood glucose to evaluate any link to hypoglycaemia. Seek medication review.

Impact on coronary heart disease risk factors	
Weight gain/increased appetite **This causes:** ◆ **failure to respond to oral anti-diabetic drugs** ◆ **worsening diabetes** ◆ **increased risk of cardiovascular disease** **In type 2 diabetes, the extra weight is mainly central adipose tissue** **Metformin may cause anorexia**	Monitor appetite, intake, weight and girth closely. Patients should record weight weekly, at same time of day, after voiding, using the same scale, in similar clothes. Waist circumference (measured above the iliac crest) should be less than 88cm (35 inches) in women, 102cm (40 inches) in men. If weight or girth increase, record dietary intake. Avoid high doses of sulphonylureas.
Lipid profile deterioration	Check lipid profile pre-therapy and regularly. Assess overall risk of coronary heart disease.

148

Heart failure **Oedema (14% patients), fluid retention, with thiazolidinediones, particularly obese patients (Kahn *et al.* 2006)** **Acarbose causes oedema very rarely**	Monitor patients for any swelling, breathlessness, or rapidly increasing weight and report to prescriber (see beta blockers). Increased vigilance if NSAIDs are co-prescribed. Thiazolidinediones are contra-indicated with insulin (BNF 2007).
Anaemia **Thiazolidinediones only**	Check full blood count pre-therapy. Pre-existing anaemia is likely to worsen.

Fluid and electrolyte disturbance

Lactic acidosis (rare, but very serious) **Metformin only** **Signs and symptoms:** ◆ **severe muscle pain** ◆ **weakness** ◆ **fatigue** ◆ **sleepiness** ◆ **rapid, shallow breathing** ◆ **gastrointestinal disturbances.**	Metformin is not administered to patients with conditions predisposing to hypoxia and lactic acid formation (see cautions). Ask patients to report signs and symptoms. If the patient develops a fever, dehydration, sepsis, urinary tract infection or a cardiovascular event, seek urgent medical advice regarding administration (Nisbet *et al.* 2004). Avoid dieting, prolonged fasting. If diabetes is worsening, seek medication review. Check serum creatinine and creatinine clearance (chapter 21): pre-therapy; during illness or suspected dehydration; if anti-hypertensives, diuretics or NSAIDs are co-prescribed; regularly (quarterly for older people or those at risk) (BNF 2007). Ensure the anaesthetic team are aware of metformin administration.
Hyponatraemia (glossary) with chlorpropamide, glipizide, glimepiride (see SIADH, antidepressants)	Report any swelling or breathlessness to prescriber. Check serum sodium concentration. Particular caution if diuretics co-administered.

Gastrointestinal disturbances

Nausea, vomiting, diarrhoea **These often limit the dose of metformin or acrabose that can be tolerated** **Metallic taste with metformin, sulphonylureas**	Metformin: administer with meals to reduce nausea; when initiating therapy, increase dose gradually. Problems may ameliorate within weeks. Acarbose: start with low doses, once daily; gradually increase to 3 times/day; avoid foods containing sucrose (confectionery).
Heartburn with sulphonylureas	Antacids unlikely to help.

149

Reduced absorption of vitamin B$_{12}$ and folates with long-term metformin Increased plasma homocysteine concentrations, which increases risks of atherosclerosis	Discuss monitoring and possible supplementation with prescriber (Davis 2006).

Genito-urinary system

Menstruation may resume (mainly women with polycystic ovaries who lose weight when treated with metformin)	Advise that improved responsiveness to insulin may restore fertility and contraceptive advice may be necessary.
Impotence or haematuria with pioglitazone	Ask patient to report these problems.

Hypersensitivity responses

Liver disorders: Acarbose	Monitor liver function pre-therapy and for first 6–12 months of therapy. If any abnormalities persist, the drug will be withdrawn.
Thiazolidinediones	Monitor liver function pre-therapy, regularly thereafter and if symptoms arise. Therapy will be withdrawn if abnormalities persist or if jaundice appears.
Meglitinides, sulphonylureas (rarely)	Report any signs or symptoms of liver failure: nausea, fatigue, upper abdominal pain, dark urine, jaundice.
Rash	Report skin reactions promptly, as they may worsen.
Photosensitivity (sunburn) Glipizide, glibenclamide, chlorpropamide	Advise patients of increased risks of sunburn, and importance of covering skin appropriately.

Therapeutic failure or persistent hyperglycaemia is relatively common

Primary failure, that is, no improvement in haemoglobin A$_{1c}$ and blood glucose concentration on initiation of therapy	Monitor haemoglobin A$_{1c}$ and blood glucose concentrations to determine treatment response (NICE 2002). Absorption may be decreased if the patient is hyperglycaemic. Thiazolidinediones may take several weeks to exert their full effects. If prescribed, acarbose should be administered in conjunction with high fibre diet, to maximise effectiveness. Discuss, with prescriber, alternative or additional therapy.

Secondary failure i.e. medication becomes less effective with time, despite compliance	Monitor progress of diabetes regularly, including glucose concentrations, lipid profile, assessment of cardiovascular system, kidneys, eyes, healing. If problems persist, insulin may be prescribed. Particular vigilance if thiazolidinediones are initiated. Higher doses of sulphonylureas confer little additional benefit.
Severe hyperglycaemia, particularly during illness or stress	Be prepared to administer insulin during acute illness, infection, fever, stress, trauma, surgery, myocardial infarction. Advise patients of the warning signs of hyperglycaemia: drowsiness, 'not coping', anorexia, nausea, abdominal pain, increased urination and thirst.

Rare adverse effects include: bone marrow suppression (chapter 21), pancreatitis.

Cautions and contra-indications:

- **Impaired renal function.** Some sulphonylureas and meglitinides may be prescribed at reduced doses: blood glucose monitoring essential.
- **Metformin:** avoid if patient is dehydrated, prescribed diuretics, shocked or creatinine clearance below 60ml/min. (ABPI 2007 Glucophage® data sheet) or 70ml/min. and serum creatinine >110 micromol/l in women and >135 micromol/l in men (ABPI 2007 Avandament® data sheet).
- **Moderate renal impairment:** avoid acarbose.
- **Severe renal impairment:** avoid thiazolidinediones.
- **Liver impairment.** Small doses of sulphonylureas may be prescribed: blood glucose monitoring essential. Avoid metformin, acarbose, nateglinide, thiazolidinediones.
- **Heart failure** precludes administration of thiazolidinediones or metformin.
- **Respiratory failure, anaemia or vascular disease** increase the risk of lactic acidosis with metformin.
- **Inflammatory bowel disease, chronic intestinal disorders.** Acarbose increases intestinal gas formation.
- **Malnourished** patients require reduced doses. Metformin is less suitable for patients who fast for prolonged periods or adopt restrictive diets.
- **Hypothyroidism,** Addison's disease may increase the risk of hypoglycaemia.
- **Pregnancy and breastfeeding.** Oral hypoglycaemics are unsuitable for women who are planning pregnancy, pregnant or breastfeeding (see insulin).
- **Children** with diabetes usually receive insulin. Metformin is occasionally prescribed by specialists.
- **Porphyria:** avoid sulphonylureas.

Interactions:

Alcohol increases the risks of **hypoglycaemia**, and should never be taken without food, or in excess of 2–3 drinks/day.

◆ Sweet drinks are best avoided.

◆ Due to the risk of lactic acidosis, manufacturers of **metformin** advise total abstinence, including alcohol-containing medicines and mouthwashes (ABPI 2007). Binge drinking, drinking without food or with liver impairment is dangerous.

◆ Some patients taking sulphonylureas, particularly chlorpropamide, experience **flushing** 5–20 minutes after drinking. If this is troublesome, an alternative sulphonylurea can be prescribed.

Metformin should be discontinued before administration of iodinated contrast agents and not re-administered for 48 hours after discontinuation, due to risk of lactic acidosis. Co-administration of NSAIDs, ACE inhibitors, diuretics, nifedipine, trimethoprim, digoxin, cimetidine may be hazardous (Aronson 2006).

Acarbose should not be co-administered with enzyme preparations and orlistat. Acarbose impairs the absorption of digoxin.

Careful monitoring is required for co-administration with:

◆ Drugs predisposing to **hyperglycaemia** or worsening diabetes, including: diuretics, thyroid hormones, amphetamines, cocaine, salbutamol, terbutaline, large quantities of caffeine, growth hormone, oestrogens and progestogens, phenothiazines, olanzapine, clozapine, corticosteroids, danazol, calcium channel blockers, some NSAIDs, some cytotoxic agents, marijuana, cigarettes, medicines containing sugar.

◆ Drugs predisposing to **hypoglycaemia,** including: insulin, additional oral anti-diabetic drugs, antifungal agents, monoamine oxidise inhibitors, ACE inhibitors, salicylates (effects usually minimal), naproxen, other NSAIDs, anabolic steroids, some antibiotics, cimetidine (rarely ranitidine), gemfibrozil (contra-indicated with meglitinides), warfarin (sulphonylureas only).

◆ Beta blockers may mask the warning signs of hypoglycaemia (see insulin).

18 Thyroid and anti-thyroid drugs

Actions: Thyroid hormones (T4 and T3) control metabolic rate and affect most body systems. Abnormal concentrations of thyroid hormones cause problems with body temperature, the nervous system, the heart, fertility, growth and development.

Indications: Both underactivity and overactivity of the thyroid are managed by medication.

♦ If the thyroid is underactive (hypothyroidism), replacement therapy is prescribed, usually levothyroxine sodium.

♦ If the thyroid is overactive (hyperthyroidism), formation of thyroid hormones can be suppressed by carbimazole or propylthiouracil.

The need for medication is assessed by clinical examination and thyroid function tests (TFTs). Blood tests are usually organised 2 weeks before patients' appointments, so that results are available. TFTs may be affected by liver or kidney function, use of salicylates, androgens, corticosteroids, amiodarone, phenytoin; this information should be included on laboratory forms.

Thyroid hormones

Administration: Levothyroxine sodium, a form of thyroxine or tetraiodothyronine (T4), is administered orally, once daily, before breakfast. Food, dietary fibre, some soy products, antacids and mineral supplements can decrease absorption. Advise patients to find a suitable routine for administration; therapy is usually lifelong. Therapy is initiated with low doses, particularly in older people, and increased every 4 weeks, as needed. Higher doses may be prescribed by specialists for thyroid suppression therapy. For infants and children, the dose is initially based on weight, and adjusted to meet the demands of growth and development.

Liothyronine is a form of triiodothyronine (T3), prescribed for severely hypothyroid patients. It acts more rapidly and is 5 times more powerful than levothyroxine.

Adverse effects:

The commonest adverse effects of thyroid hormone therapy are the signs and symptoms of hyperthyroidism, caused by **excessive doses**. Problems may take 3–5 weeks to develop and persist 1–3 weeks after dose reduction.

Cardiovascular problems may occur without other features of hyperthyroidism, particularly in those >50. Thyroid hormones increase metabolic rate, heart rate, and cardiac output. Therefore the heart has to work harder and needs more oxygen (Box 6.1). If the coronary arteries are narrowed, they may not be able to deliver extra oxygen. Shortage of oxygen causes angina, cardiac dysrhythmia or heart failure.

If doses are too low the signs and symptoms of hypothyroidism develop. Even small changes in the dose of thyroxine may make a significant change in metabolic rate and energy expenditure. Thyroid hormones are essential for the breakdown of cholesterol. Increased cholesterol concentration is an early sign of hypothyroidism.

Other body systems: thyroid hormones affect mood and behaviour, metabolic rate and gastrointestinal function. New patients presenting to mental health services have thyroid function tests as routine screening.

Adverse effects: implications for practice: LEVOTHYROXINE SODIUM

Regular follow up, assessment and blood tests are essential. When the patient is stabilised, annual appointments may be sufficient.

Potential Problem	Suggestions for Prevention and Management
Excessive doses	
Cardiovascular problems	
Tachycardia	Instruct patients to check radial pulse weekly.
	If resting pulse is above 85–100bpm or irregular, withhold next dose and seek medical advice.
Chest pain caused by myocardial ischaemia	ECG pre-therapy and follow up.
	Therapy is initiated cautiously, and evaluated regularly.
	If patients report chest pain, withhold and inform prescriber. Dosage reduction may be necessary.
	Ensure anaesthetic teams are informed of medication.
	Advise 'medi-alert' identification.
Cardiac dysrhythmia causing palpitations or syncope (fainting)	Monitor radial pulse and apex beat, simultaneously to detect atrial fibrillation.
	Check BP and ECG.
	Arrange ECG if irregularities detected.
Heart failure, poor exercise tolerance	Careful assessment (see beta blockers) and individualised dosage adjustments.
Neurological problems	
Tremor	Ask patient to stretch out hands and fingers to assess any tremor.
	Inquire about difficulties with activities, such as writing.
Restlessness, excitability, irritability, short temper, hypomania/mania Interpersonal skills and relationships may be affected	Advise patient to report these problems as they may indicate that dosage is excessive. Arrange thyroid function tests (TFTs).

Insomnia	Administer levothyroxine first thing in the morning.
Gastrointestinal function is affected by thyroid status	
Diarrhoea Nausea	Contact prescriber if bowel movements become more frequent than 3/day or if nausea develops.
Increased absorption of glucose. Hyperglycaemia within the first 2 hours after a meal	Check blood glucose on initiation of therapy and during medication review. Advise patients with diabetes to monitor glucose. Be prepared to increase insulin doses.
Increased metabolic rate in all tissues	
Pyrexia, heat intolerance, sweating, flushing Muscle cramp or weakness	Arrange TFTs and report to prescriber.
Weight loss despite increased appetite	Record weight weekly.
Hair loss	Usually reverses as thyroid function normalises.
Increased risk of osteoporosis	No (or minimal) extra risk if thyroid status remains normal. Patients receiving suppression therapy may need protection against osteoporosis, for example a diet with high quantities of calcium and vitamin D (see corticosteroids).
Underdose of levothyroxine	
Tiredness, constipation, excessive menstrual loss, weight gain, depression In older people: incontinence, stumbling/falling, cold intolerance, 'dementia', hair loss, dry skin	Assess patient. Monitor TFTs and serum cholesterol, which should be within normal range. Emollients may help dry skin. Extra vigilance for pressure areas. Consider compliance aids. Dosage requirements increase during serious illness, such as pneumonia, stroke, heart failure; arrange TFTs.
On initiation of therapy	
Diabetes and adrenal disorders may be unmasked	Obtain venous blood samples to assess glucose and electrolytes.
Diuresis for a few days	Warn patients. Ensure access to facilities.
Therapeutic failure	
Slow initial response The half-life (glossary) of thyroxine is about 7 days,	Advise that it may take 4–6 weeks for benefits to be experienced. Arrange TFTs 4–6 weeks after each change of dose.

and full effects will not be achieved for 5 weeks. In addition, as metabolic rate increases, the rate of hormone clearance increases, and higher doses may be needed	Skin and hair texture may not return to a healthy 'normal' for 6 months. Consider drug interactions (below).
Blood tests are within the normal range, but patient continues to feel unwell	Consider referral to specialist for consideration of regimen change, such as addition of liothyronine (Gitlin *et al.* 2004, Aronson 2006).

Allergic reactions to levothyroxine are very rare.

Cautions and contra-indications:

♦ Older people, particularly with pre-existing **cardiovascular disorders**. Patients aged >50 receive lower initial doses, and more gradual increments. Patients awaiting cardiac surgery may defer replacement therapy.

♦ If hypothyroidism has gone undiagnosed for a long time, adverse reactions are more likely; therefore, initial and incremental doses are lower.

♦ Disorders of the pituitary or adrenal complicate management. Seek specialist advice.

♦ Diabetes may be worsened.

♦ Pregnancy. Specialist care should be sought at the earliest opportunity as blood tests and dose increases are often needed within the first trimester (Glinoer & Abalovich 2007).

♦ Breastfeeding is regarded as safe.

♦ Children receiving thyroid replacement therapy have growth and development monitored in specialist centres.

♦ Missed doses. Avoid administering 2 doses close together. If therapy is suspended for >7 days, symptoms of hypothyroidism are likely to appear.

Interactions (summary): Advise patients to inform all prescribers of thyroid hormone therapy and to seek advice from pharmacists before buying non-prescription products.

♦ Salbutamol, terbutaline, ketamine, dopamine, adrenaline/epinephrine, 'cold cures', amphetamines and cocaine increase the risk of cardiac problems.

♦ Tricyclic antidepressants may increase the risk of cardiac dysrhythmias or alter thyroid function.

♦ Warfarin. Anticoagulant dose may need reduction. Monitor blood clotting closely, particularly 4–6 weeks after changes in thyroid hormone dose.

♦ Oestrogens increase the dose requirements.

♦ Some antiepileptic drugs, rifampicin, some antimalarials and sertraline may reduce, and some antiviral drugs may increase, effects of therapy. Thyroid function should be monitored carefully (McCowen *et al.* 1997).

♦ Digoxin and theophylline dose requirements vary according to thyroid status.

♦ Thyroid status may be altered by: lithium, quetiapine, amiodarone, interferon beta.

♦ Some drugs, such as sodium polystyrene sulphonate and cimetidine, reduce absorption of thyroid hormones. Administration of sucralfate, cholestyramine, iron, calcium, magnesium or aluminium compounds (including some antacids) should be separated from thyroid hormones by 4 hours (Baxter 2006).

Anti-thyroid drugs

Actions and indications: Anti-thyroid drugs interfere with the synthesis of thyroid hormones. They may be prescribed to manage the signs and symptoms of hyperthyroidism until the disease remits of its own accord or in conjunction with other treatments (Abraham *et al.* 2003, Farwell & Braverman 2006).

Administration: Carbimazole is administered orally, at regular intervals, with a consistent relation to meals (ABPI 2007). Inform patients that signs and symptoms will not be relieved until the existing thyroid hormones have been eliminated from the body, which takes some 1–6 weeks, depending on severity of hyperthyroidism. Beta blockers may be co-prescribed to control symptoms during this time. Propylthiouracil is usually reserved for patients who react adversely to carbimazole.

Adverse effects: implications for practice:

CARBIMAZOLE

Potential Problem	Suggestions for Prevention and Management
Hypothyroidism, from excessive doses	
Tiredness, constipation, excessive menstrual loss, weight gain, depression **In older people: incontinence, stumbling/ falling, cold intolerance, 'dementia', hair loss, dry skin**	Regular review is essential, particularly 7 weeks after initiation of therapy, when maximum effect is experienced. Monitor for hypothyroidism, as above.
Compliance. Patients complain of slowness, lethargy and weight gain, despite normal blood test results. This leads to non-compliance	Advise that, initially, these problems are common when long-standing hyperthyroidism is corrected. Many patients are underweight on diagnosis; advise that weight may 'normalise'.
Gastrointestinal disturbances, often mild	Nausea usually subsides within weeks. Administer with meals to reduce nausea.

Loss of sense of taste	In older people, ensure this does not impair nutritional status. Monitor intake.
Hypersensitivity responses	
Bone marrow suppression can arise abruptly: ♦ **Agranulocytosis (seriously low white cell count), 0.03% of patients** ♦ **pancytopenia (anaemia, low platelets, low white cells), rarer** **Higher risk in first months of therapy**	Ask patients to report the first indication of sore throat, mouth ulcers, pyrexia, bruising and non-specific signs of infection. Immediate full blood count and inform prescriber. Withhold therapy until results available. If condition is confirmed, liaise with specialists, urgently.
Mild reduction in white cell count	This is not clinically important.
Rashes, itching may be associated with serious allergies	Report. Prescriber may substitute propylthiouracil. If itching is due to dry skin, this may indicate hypothyroidism.
Bone and joint pain **Muscle pain**	These may subside within 2–3 weeks. Check creatine phosphokinase concentrations in venous blood sample.
Jaundice, liver and pancreatic disorders (rare)	Prescriber may withhold therapy until investigations are complete. Monitor liver function if patients are prescribed propylthiouracil after adverse reaction to carbimazole.
Therapeutic failure	
Persistent hyperthyroidism	After 7–8 weeks, other treatment options may be explored with specialists. Illness and infection may affect dosage requirements. Dividing the dose of carbimazole and maintaining a constant relationship between medication and meals may improve disease control.
Relapse, following remission	It is prudent to avoid all preparations containing iodine and drugs affecting the thyroid (below), wherever possible.

Rare side effects include peripheral nerve damage, vasculitis and (reversible) hair loss.

Cautions and contra-indications (carbimazole):

◆ Liver disorders.

◆ Bone marrow abnormalities.

◆ Previous hypersensitivity to any anti-thyroid drugs.

◆ Pregnancy. Specialists prescribe the lowest doses needed to keep the woman euthyroid.

◆ Breastfeeding. Manufacturers advise avoid.

◆ Children. Seek specialist advice.

Interactions: carbimazole (summary):

Co-administration of other drugs suppressing the bone marrow, for example, clozapine, anti-cancer drugs, increase the risk of serious adverse reactions.

Response to carbimazole may be altered by: preparations or vitamins containing iodine, such as kelp, certain contrast media, topical povidone iodine; drugs affecting the thyroid, including amiodarone, lithium, sulphonamides, interferons, possibly phenytoin and quetiapine.

Warfarin, prednisolone and digoxin doses may need adjusting as thyroid status changes.

Erythromycin may be best avoided (Koh 2001).

Smoking may worsen the ophthalmological complications of Graves' disease.

159

19 Cytotoxic Drugs

Cancer is a whole-body disease, in which abnormal forms of the body's cells divide, multiply and spread, uncontrolled by normal regulators. Treatments may be directed at cure, palliation or prolonging life.

Drugs prescribed to treat cancer include: cytotoxics; immunological therapies; hormones and hormone antagonists.

Actions: Cytotoxic drugs damage actively dividing cells. However, they may be unable to destroy any malignant cells which are in the 'resting' stage of the cell cycle (glossary). If these cells become active later, the immune system often cannot eliminate them. Therefore, anti-cancer therapy may be repeated in cycles, to catch any malignant cells as they emerge from their 'resting' state. With each cycle, a proportion of actively dividing cells is killed. Therefore, several cycles of therapy are often needed. However, patients who experience severe adverse drug reactions in early cycles, may decline further treatments and consequently adverse reactions should be promptly and effectively managed.

Cytotoxic drugs are usually divided into:

- ◆ alkylating drugs e.g. cyclophosphamide, chlorambucil.
- ◆ cytotoxic antibiotics e.g. doxorubicin, bleomycin.
- ◆ antimetabolites e.g. methotrexate, cytarabine, cladribine.
- ◆ vinca alkaloids (e.g. vincristine) and etoposide.
- ◆ other anti-neoplastic drugs, including: platinum compounds (e.g. cisplatin, carboplatin); taxanes; and others.

Some cytotoxic drugs act on discrete stages of cell division. Others act on all stages of the cell cycle, but not cells in the 'resting' state e.g. cisplatin, cyclophosphamide. Other drugs, such as bleomycin, kill cells in the resting phase, but are more active against all actively dividing cells (Rang et al. 2007). Cytotoxics are often administered together. Combination therapy may be more toxic than monotherapy but this is balanced against enhanced response, reduced development of drug resistance and increased survival.

Immunotherapy includes: immunosuppressants, such as azathioprine, ciclosporin; corticosteroids, monoclonal antibodies, interferons.

Hormonal therapy is employed in treatment of breast, uterine and prostate cancers. For example, anti-oestrogen treatments, such as tamoxifen, increase breast cancer survival rates.

Indications and administration: Anti-cancer drugs may be prescribed alone or together with surgery or radiotherapy. They may be prescribed before surgery to shrink tumours, or post-operatively, to destroy any remaining cancer cells.

Administration is guided by local and national protocols (BNF 2007, Dougherty 2004). Preparation and administration of intravenous drugs must be under carefully controlled conditions. Tablets should never be crushed, or capsules opened. Any skin or mucous membrane contact must be treated urgently with prolonged washing, according to established protocols.

Doses are calculated by specialists in relation to the patient's condition, therapeutic regimen, age, liver and kidney function, weight and (sometimes) height or body surface area. Recording weight and height on drug charts facilitates surface area calculations.

Adverse effects:

◆ those occurring with most cytotoxics: impaired cell division; excess cell breakdown.

◆ those restricted to specific agents.

Most cytotoxics

Cell division impeded: Malignant cells are similar to normal cells. Therefore, cytotoxics also kill dividing cells in healthy tissue, causing severe side effects, and limiting the efficacy of treatment. Impaired cell division affects:

◆ **Gastrointestinal system.** The cells lining the gut are actively dividing. Cytotoxic drugs inhibit this cell division, thinning the protective layers and rendering the lining fragile. The normal microflora may invade the tissues, for example causing severe thrush. **Emesis** and anorexia also arise from central actions of drugs and products of cell breakdown on the vomiting centre (Figure 12.1).

◆ **Bone marrow** contains the most actively dividing cells of the body in the non-pregnant adult. All drugs which affect cell division will reduce production of white cells, red cells and platelets. The immune system may become disabled, and unable to cope with infections or the normal microflora. Another function of the immune system is to protect the body from cancer. Cancer treatment may reduce the effectiveness of the body's 'cancer surveillance' system, and further cancers may arise in survivors.

◆ **Skin and mucous membranes.** All lining tissues, including the epidermis and hair, are continuously being renewed by cell division in the basal layer of the skin. If this is impaired, the skin becomes thin and more vulnerable to injury, including that from UV light.

◆ **Healing.** The cells responsible for forming new tissue, the fibroblasts (glossary), are unable to multiply. Therefore, formation of new proteins, such as collagen, is compromised.

◆ **Growth and reproduction.** Formation of reproductive cells (gametes) and body growth requires normal cell division.

◆ **Cell breakdown excessive.** Uric acid is formed as cells are broken down by anti-cancer agents. The enzymes which normally convert it to harmless urea may be overwhelmed by the quantity of uric acid liberated. Therefore, plasma concentration of uric acid may increase, and may cause gout.

Adverse effects: implications for practice: CYTOTOXICS

Many of the problems below are common to most therapeutic regimens. Problems confined to certain drugs are indicated.

Potential Problem	Suggestions for Prevention and Management
Gastrointestinal disturbance	
Emesis See Table 12.1	Ensure preventive anti-emetic therapy is administered for acute, delayed and anticipatory symptoms. Eliminate unpleasant smells from environment. Ensure oral hygiene is optimal and ice cubes are available. Serve meals at room temperature. Advise resting for 1–2 hours after meals. Mobilise gradually. Avoid sudden head movements, for example when transferring the patient. Allow extra time for mobilising.
Anorexia	Monitor intake. Offer small frequent meals of patient's choice. Separate drinks and fruits from meals by 30–60 minutes, if possible. Ensure food is available any time patients are hungry. Offer high-calorie foods, such as cream and whole milk. Cold food may be more palatable than hot food.
Bitter taste	If patient refuses meat, due to bitter taste, offer alternative protein, such as dairy products. Plastic cutlery may help.
Oral Mucositis (breakdown of lining of mouth and oesophagus) Highest risk at 5–10 days after initiation Particularly fluorouracil, methotrexate, doxorubicin and related compounds	Prevention is more effective than treatment. Instigate mouth care at earliest opportunity. Suggest hourly rinses with water. Use soft toothbrushes 2–3 times/day. Avoid abrasive, hot or spicy food, vinegar and smoking. Inspect the oral cavity regularly for early signs of damage. Avoid ill-fitting dentures. Sucking ice during fluorouracil infusions may help.
Folinic acid derivatives, such as calcium folinate, may be prescribed with methotrexate or fluorouracil	Observe for possible hypersensitivity responses and fever.
Mucositis of bowel causing diarrhoea	Monitor bowel movements and fluid loss. Check electrolytes. Ensure perianal area is scrupulously clean. Avoid enemas, if possible, as they may injure the bowel wall. Avoid large meals and foods causing flatulence, such as beans

and cabbage. Ensure dietary advice does not lead to constipation.

Monitor patient for systemic infection, caused by gastrointestinal organisms crossing the damaged gut wall.

Bone marrow suppression: 7–10 days after initiation or later with alkylating agents	
1. Low white cell count/ neutropenia. Severe or life-threatening infection may follow **Recovery usually occurs after some 21 days** **Folinic acid derivatives may be prescribed (above)**	Monitor full blood counts regularly. If results are abnormal, doctors may decide to delay treatment. Monitor for infection, for example, raised body temperature 4–6.00pm. Ask patient to report any sore throat, chills, burning urine, cough. Adopt aseptic techniques. Avoid catheters, where possible. Advise patient to avoid exposure to infection, particularly days 7–10 of therapy. Discuss any associated social isolation.
Filgrastim and related 'colony stimulating factors' may be prescribed	Monitor possible adverse reactions, including gastrointestinal disturbance, muscle pain, headache, painful urination, reactions at injection site, lung damage, hypersensitivity responses.
Further cancers, for example, leukaemia associated with alkylating agents (BNF 2007). Risks may be up to 6 times greater than in the general population	Life-long cancer surveillance for survivors (Aronson 2006).
2. Anaemia may be severe and cause incapacitating tiredness	Review diet and nutritional supplements. If erythropoietins are prescribed, monitor for possible hypertension, and to ensure that haemoglobin concentration remains below 12g/dL.
Fatigue, may be profound. It may be due to disease or treatment	Check full blood count. Ensure adequate intake. Advise frequent rests. Plan activities, including holidays, if possible.
3. Low platelet count, causing bruising and bleeding **If constipation arises, straining at stool may cause rectal bleeding**	Check platelets and report problems. Monitor stools and urine for blood. If shaving is essential, use electric razors. Avoid suppositories, rectal thermometers, intramuscular injections if possible. Monitor bowel motions.

Skin and mucous membranes	
Injuries	Pressure area vigilance.
	Avoid friction and shearing forces (see corticosteroids).
	Allow extra time for procedures such as transfer to hoist, care of infusion sites.
	Administer skin care and emollients.
Increased risk of sunburn (see antipsychotics)	Advise dark glasses and covering skin with clothing and sunscreen during exposure to direct sunlight.
Hair loss/alopecia **Alteration of body image may be associated** **Hair usually returns some 8 weeks after therapy, but may be of different colour or texture**	Wash and comb hair very gently. Use wide-tooth combs. Suggest silk pillows. Protect hair from the wind. If hair loss occurs, ensure head covering is available to prevent sunburn or excess loss of body heat. Select a wig of the patient's own hair colour, preferably before loss.
Dryness of vagina	Refer to specialists. Vaginal gel may be prescribed to prevent dyspareunia.
Impaired healing	Anticipate poor healing and contact wound care specialists promptly. Take swabs if healing delayed.
Growth and reproduction	
Infertility/sterility **Premature menopause** **(Particularly alkylating agents)**	If the patient's family is not considered complete, refer to specialists promptly regarding storage of reproductive cells or tissue. (Broaching this with teenagers who have just received a diagnosis of cancer requires a high level of communication skills.)
Impaired growth in children	Monitor growth and encourage optimum nutrition. Liaise with multidisciplinary team regarding education and adequate intellectual stimulation.
Accumulation of uric acid	
Kidney damage and gout	Ensure uric acid is monitored in venous blood samples. Report joint or neck pain. If allopurinol or rasburicase are prescribed, monitor for possible side effects, such as gastrointestinal and allergy problems.
Hypersensitivity responses	
Skin reactions, fever, chills and anaphylaxis	Report rashes to prescriber. Ensure protocols are in place for emergency management.

Therapeutic failure	
May be caused by patient non-compliance	Minimise adverse effects, particularly nausea, as much as possible. Customised patient education to achieve concordance may help. Monitor compliance after discharge.

Toxicity associated with specific cytotoxics:

More rarely, certain drugs damage various organs of the body.

Potential Problem	**Suggestions for Prevention and Management**
Kidney damage **methotrexate, cisplatin**	Monitor fluid balance and/or standardised daily weights. Ensure patient is always well hydrated. Recommend daily fluid intake of 35ml/kg body weight for adults (120ml/kg for infants), including several glasses of water. Offer a selection of cool, clear liquids.
Haemorrhagic cystitis (extremely painful) cyclophophamide and related drugs	Encourage fluids for 24–48 hours after administration. If mesna is prescribed, be aware of possible emetic and other side effects.
Heart damage **Dysrhythmia – early** **Heart failure – late** **Doxorubicin, daunorubicin** **Infants and older people most vulnerable**	Monitor cardiovascular system, vital signs, breathlessness, ECG, if indicated.
Nerve damage **Vincristine, vinblastine, cisplatin, oxaliplatin** **Complete recovery may take months**	Report abdominal pain, constipation, burning pain, numbness or loss of function in limbs or fingers.
Confusion, coma mainly high dose alkylating agents	Guard against falls in older people.
Hearing loss mainly cisplatin	Test hearing during therapy.
Lung damage **bleomycin, doxorubicin, methotrexate, alkylating agents (rarely)**	Pre-therapy and follow-up chest X ray and lung function tests.

Extravasation from intravenous lines:
Not all cytotoxics damage tissues e.g. bleomycin, cyclophosphamide. Most cause inflammation, while others e.g. doxorubicin, vinca alkaloids, cause blistering and necrosis.
Protocols for managing extravasation vary with drug administered and whether central or peripheral lines are used. Detailed information on antidotes and protocols is available in Aronson (2006): Cytotoxic and immunosuppressant drugs.

Severe tissue damage, requiring plastic surgery, has been reported	Ensure line is patent by administering another solution before the drug.
	Check site frequently.
	Ask patients to report any discomfort.
	Stop infusion immediately extravasation is suspected, but leave line in place.
	Ensure antidotes are available; depending on the drug, warm or cold packs, sodium thiosulphate or hyaluronidase may be required.

Cautions and contra-indications:

◆ **Impaired liver or kidney function** may necessitate dose reduction. Kidney function, and, consequently, ability to eliminate drugs, may change during therapy. Therefore, prescribers will require regular assessments of serum creatinine and glomerular filtration rate (chapter 21).

◆ **Dehydration** (from vomiting, diarrhoea, hypercalcaemia) may necessitate postponement of treatment.

◆ **Pregnancy.** Pregnant staff (and those who may be pregnant) should not handle cytotoxics. Patients should be advised to use effective barrier contraception, if appropriate. Many anti-cancer drugs can damage the fetus or cause miscarriage. If cancer is diagnosed during pregnancy, the woman is confronted with very difficult decisions.

◆ **Breastfeeding** is contra-indicated.

◆ **Children.** If physical isolation is necessary to reduce exposure to infection, discuss measures to minimise social isolation.

◆ **Older patients** are more vulnerable to adverse effects, as they have reduced bone marrow, cardiac and renal reserves.

◆ **Immunisations** may be ineffective. If live vaccines, such as BCG, MMR are administered, vaccine-related illness may develop. Administration should be delayed at least 6 months after treatment (DH 2006).

◆ **Disposal of patients' body fluids/secretions** should follow local protocols, during treatment and for at least a further 48 hours. Gloves should be worn. Most anti-cancer drugs are metabolised to inactive forms before being secreted in urine or faeces (Dougherty 2004).

Interactions: Patients should seek advice before taking any non-prescription drugs, e.g. cimetidine, aspirin and alcohol. Many non-steroidal anti-inflammatory drugs can reduce the excretion of methotrexate and thus increase the risk of toxicity. Effectiveness of etoposide may be reduced by St John's Wort.

Anti-cancer drugs interact with many other drugs. Co-administration with other drugs which adversely affect bone marrow, such as clozapine, may increase the risk of neutropenia. Other examples include:

◆ If oxygen >30% is given to patients taking bleomycin, there is a risk of serious lung damage.

◆ Mercaptopurine absorption is decreased by food.

◆ Methotrexate mucositis may be increased by nitrous oxide, for example used for dressing changes.

◆ Cyclophosphamide and related drugs enhance the actions of suxamethonium (a muscle relaxant administered before surgery).

Contributors

John Knight BSc, PhD. Lecturer, School of Health Science, Swansea University

Janet Jones RN, MSc, BEd, RNT. Lecturer in Cancer Nursing (retired), School of Health Sciences, Swansea University

20 Non-Steroidal Anti-Inflammatory Drugs (NSAIDs)

NSAIDs reduce inflammation, pain, fever and clotting, mainly by inhibiting the formation of prostaglandins, which are important mediators of pain and inflammation in the tissues and of temperature control in the hypothalamus.

NSAIDs include the traditional agents, such as aspirin, ibuprofen, diclofenac, naproxen, piroxicam, indometacin and the newer cyclo-oxygenase-2 (COX2) inhibitors, such as celecoxib, etoricoxib. Paracetamol (acetaminophen in the USA) is similar to the NSAIDs, but is not anti-inflammatory (below).

Actions: Prostaglandins are formed when cell membranes are disturbed, for example by invading micro-organisms, tissue damage, allergy, or other conditions. An important enzyme in this process is cyclo-oxygenase. The key action of NSAIDs is to block the action of this enzyme and reduce the synthesis of prostaglandins. Thus, NSAIDs reduce the build-up of this important group of pain mediators, and prevent pain and inflammation. However, NSAIDs do not block the pain mediators that are already formed in the tissues, so they are less effective at relieving pain than they are at preventing it.

NSAIDs not only block prostaglandin formation, they also interfere with related compounds responsible for clotting (the thromboxanes) and blood flow (the prostacyclins). Therefore, NSAIDs not only reduce pain and inflammation, but also affect the clotting mechanisms and the blood supply to vital organs, including gut and kidney. This can have deleterious consequences, particularly in the long term and in older people.

Paracetamol acts on the same enzymes, but only in the central nervous system.

Indications:

◆ NSAIDs are used for pain, inflammation, and fever. They control symptoms in: musculo-skeletal disorders, including rheumatoid arthritis; injury; migraine; headaches; dysmenorrhoea; dental pain; post-operative pain.

◆ Control of fever (paracetamol), particularly patients with epilepsy or fever >40°C.

◆ Prevention of cardiovascular and cerebrovascular thrombosis (aspirin). Lower dose than prescribed for pain relief.

◆ Management of a cardiac ischaemic event: 150–300mg aspirin chewed or dispersed in water.

Administration:

◆ NSAIDs are more effective at preventing than relieving pain. When pain is anticipated, doses should be administered at regular intervals. How often the drug is administered depends on guidelines for each drug and on the patient's needs: for example, some patients may find that ibuprofen 3 times a day is adequate, whereas other patients on the same regimen will experience 'break through' pain before the next dose and require 4 doses each day.

◆ Most NSAIDs are taken orally, with or after meals, accompanied by a full glass of water or milk. Remain upright 30 minutes after ingestion. Slow-release preparations offer few advantages and are more likely to damage the lower gastrointestinal tract. Orodispersible or liquid preparations may offer more rapid pain relief.

◆ Suppositories may be absorbed erratically and/or cause rectal irritation, ulceration or stenosis (Box 1.2).

◆ Topical preparations are applied in the direction of the hair follicles. Irritation may be caused by application over shaved areas.

◆ Intravenous and intra-muscular preparations are available. For example, for up to 2 days, diclofenac may be administered by intravenous infusion (not bolus) or intra-muscular injection deep into the gluteal muscle (Figures 10.1, 10.2), using alternate sides. Patients report that this is very painful. Administer only clear solutions.

◆ NSAIDs reduce pain and fever rapidly (within an hour), but take up to 3 weeks to reduce inflammation. The duration of analgesia depends on the individual drug and the patient. Generally, older patients eliminate drugs more slowly, and are vulnerable to drug accumulation. Therefore, NSAIDs with the longest duration of action, such as piroxicam, are less suitable for older people.

Adverse effects: Without prostaglandins, several systems are compromised (Jordan & White 2001).

◆ **Bleeding.** NSAIDs reduce the activity of the platelets, and thereby inhibit clotting. NSAIDs also irritate the lining of the GI tract. The risk of bleeding is related to the dose administered.

◆ **Disruption of lining of GI tract.** Prostaglandins are important in maintaining the integrity and blood supply to the lining of the gut.

◆ **Renal impairment.** Prostaglandins are important in maintaining the blood flow into the renal tubules, and the glomerular filtration rate, particularly during periods of dehydration (Figure 3.1). Any reduction in blood flow into the kidneys may lead to retention of fluid and electrolytes and a rise in blood pressure. This, in turn, can precipitate heart failure (Slordal & Spigset 2006). With long-term use, NSAIDs can also damage the kidneys and cause renal failure (Gooch *et al*. 2007).

◆ **Cardiovascular disease.** In addition to hypertension and heart failure, COX_2 inhibitors inhibit the production of prostacyclin by the blood vessels endothelial cells, and cause the vessels to narrow (Garrett & Fitzgerald 2004).

◆ **Poor healing.** Prostaglandins are integral to the natural healing processes and play a part in bone formation and turnover. NSAIDs may disrupt the formation of new blood vessels, important in healing.

◆ **Neurological effects.** NSAIDs act in the CNS to normalise body temperature. They also cause release of noradrenaline (norepinephrine), which may be responsible for the confusion sometimes observed in older patients.

◆ **Hypersensitivity responses.** When the enzyme cyclo-oxygenase is inhibited, the prostaglandin metabolic pathway is diverted to form the inflammatory mediators responsible for allergy and hypersensitivity.

Adverse effects: implications for practice:

LONG-TERM ADMINISTRATION OF NSAIDs

Although there are some differences between the NSAIDs, the risks of adverse effects are very similar at higher doses. Adverse effects may occur with all routes of administration.

Potential Problem	Suggestions for Prevention and Management
Bleeding	
Blood loss from the gastrointestinal tract The stomach is the most vulnerable organ, but enteric coated tablets can cause localised ulcers lower down the gastrointestinal tract **Extra vigilance is needed: in the first 4 weeks of therapy or increased dose; with older patients at all doses**	Serious events can occur without warning symptoms. Undertake: ◆ Full blood count before and during therapy ◆ Tests for faecal occult blood. Ibuprofen (below 1.2g/day) is probably the NSAID with lowest risk of bleeding, but paracetamol is safer. If NSAIDs cannot be withdrawn, proton-pump inhibitors or H$_2$ receptor antagonists or misoprostol (chapter 2) may be co-prescribed for high-risk patients to reduce gastric and duodenal ulceration. Warn patients that misoprostol may cause colic and/or diarrhoea.
Bleeding tendencies (particularly if other anticoagulants or corticosteroids are co-prescribed)	Check: ◆ gums for signs of bleeding ◆ skin for bruising and petechiae. Undertake: ◆ urinalysis for haematuria ◆ full blood count to detect anaemia, any folate deficiency, and platelet count ◆ assessment of prothrombin time. Ensure that the patient does not have a history of alcohol abuse or liver disease before administration. Discuss with prescriber any possible need for discontinuation before surgery/dental extraction.
Disruption of lining of gatrointestinal tract	
Gastric pain or upset, anorexia, nausea, vomiting, indigestion, stomatitis	Avoid co-administration with alcohol. In older patients, take steps to prevent malnutrition: ◆ weigh regularly ◆ monitor diet ◆ inquire about mouth soreness and denture fit. Advise that problems are exacerbated by smoking.
Protein loss	Check serum albumin.
Failure to absorb vitamin C and folates	Consider dietary supplements and serum measurements.

Management of diabetes	Monitor blood sugar and discuss with prescriber any need to reduce dose of anti-diabetic medication.
	Advise patients with diabetes taking regular aspirin to assess control by blood testing.

Kidney function, fluid balance and the cardiovascular system	
Renal impairment	Urinalysis for albuminuria/microalbuminuria.
Older people are at particular risk	Check serum creatinine and urea before and during therapy (chapter 21).
Fluid retention and risk of heart failure (particularly older adults taking ibuprofen, COX$_2$ inhibitors)	Avoid regular use of preparations containing sodium, including effervescent formulations, in the elderly e.g. Brufen® granules contain 200mg sodium (max. 4 tablets/day), Tylex® effervescent tablets contain 300mg sodium (max. 8 tablets/day) (BNF 2007). (Recommended maximum sodium intake is 2.4g/day.)
	Monitor weight.
	Ask patient to observe ankles and fingers and report swelling (see beta blockers).
	Assess cardiac insufficiency and breathlessness: inquire regarding any changes in the number of pillows used to sleep, or the ability to walk upstairs.
Hypertension **Antagonism of anti-hypertensive therapy**	Monitor blood pressure pre-therapy and regularly for patients using long-term NSAIDs or paracetamol.
Potassium retention and hyperkalaemia	Avoid potassium supplements, including those purchased in non-prescription medicines, and other drugs which increase potassium concentration (e.g. angiotensin II antagonists, ACEIs, potassium-sparing diuretics, ciclosporin) or ensure serum potassium is monitored.
Cardiovascular/ cerebrovascular disease **The increased risk of atherosclerosis and cardiovascular disorders may remain high after discontinuation**	People who use or have regularly used COX$_2$ inhibitors (for example for arthritis) should continue to be monitored for hypertension and heart failure for several years (Garrett & Fitzgerald 2004).

Disruption of Healing	
Impaired healing. The evidence that NSAIDs and COX$_2$ inhibitors may delay healing is equivocal	Monitor fractures.
	Measure wounds, including pressure sores.
	Report delayed healing.
Masking signs of infection and inflammation	Be aware of manifestations of infection, other than fever or inflammation, particularly with diabetic patients. If possible, advise paracetamol in preference to NSAIDs for patients with ulceration. Take swabs and seek advice from a wound-care specialist if wound healing is delayed.

Bone and joint damage	Use paracetamol where possible, particularly for patients with osteoarthritis.
Neurological problems	
Headache	Avoid non-prescription NSAIDs containing caffeine. Caffeine or caffeine-withdrawal may cause headaches.
Damage to inner ear	Advise patient to discontinue NSAID should tinnitus occur. This may be a warning sign that the delicate nerve cells of the inner ear are being damaged.
Confusion, dizziness, fatigue, somnolence (particularly naproxen), disturbed sleep	Advise patients to be aware of their response to NSAIDs before resuming driving or operating machinery. Alcohol will intensify any problems. Keep doses to minimum needed to manage pain.
Hypothermia following administration for fever (Nabulsi *et al.* 2005)	Monitor core body temperature if high doses of paracetamol suppositories are given to children.
Eyes	
Increased risk of epithelial damage with eye drops, due to reduced sensation of pain	Ensure patients understand that NSAID eye drops are for short-term use only.
Blurred vision and, very occasionally, serious problems have been reported	Advise patients to seek advice if discomfort occurs and to inform opticians of any NSAIDs they are taking.
Reproductive system	
Reduced fertility in women with long-term use	If long-term NSAIDs are essential for women trying to conceive, advise that this problem reverses on discontinuation.
Hypersensitivity responses	
Bronchospasm	Avoid NSAIDs in people with asthma, if possible. Monitor airways 2–3 times each day to detect early signs of worsening asthma. Prompt response to worsening asthma, difficulty breathing or a 'closing of the throat'.
Liver impairment (particularly diclofenac)	Liver function tests within 8 weeks of initiation of long-term therapy.
Anaphylactic-like reaction, with bronchospasm and cardiovascular collapse	Ensure allergies to aspirin or other NSAIDs are documented. Particular caution with people who keep bees, as reactions to stings may be worsened.

Bone marrow suppression is rare (chapter 21).

Cautions and contra-indications:

◆ **Known hypersensitivity** to aspirin, any NSAID, tartrazine or any component of an injection. A life-threatening reaction could ensue. Allergy to sulfonamides may indicate allergy to celecoxib.

◆ **Asthma**, hypertension, heart failure, epilepsy, psychotic disturbances or Parkinsonism may be worsened (particularly indometacin).

◆ **High risk of bleeding**, for example, liver failure (particularly dangerous with oesophageal varices), thrombocytopenia, vitamin K or C deficiency, peptic ulceration, haemorrhagic stroke. African Americans have a higher incidence of gastrointestinal bleeding.

◆ **Inflammatory bowel disease** may progress without recognition (particularly enteric-coated NSAIDs), due to 'masking' of symptons.

◆ **Poor renal function**: low doses may be prescribed in mild renal failure but NSAIDs (including topical applications) are contra-indicated in moderate/severe renal failure.

◆ **Heart failure** and fluid retention may be worsened. NSAIDs are contra-indicated in severe heart failure.

◆ **Hypertension** may be worsened, particularly COX_2 inhibitors.

◆ **Cardiovascular and cerebrovascular disease:** COX_2 inhibitors are contra-indicated.

◆ **Pregnancy**. Prostaglandins are important in childbirth. Use in pregnancy is associated with increased risks of bleeding, miscarriage, prolonged labour, intra-uterine growth retardation. Use in third trimester may affect fetal heart, lungs or kidneys. Paracetamol advised as an alternative, but heavy use in late pregnancy may be linked to infant wheezing.

◆ **Breastfeeding**. Increased risks of bleeding and, with aspirin, Reye's syndrome and jaundice (including topical use). Paracetamol considered safe.

◆ 8–12 days after medical termination of pregnancy with misoprostol and mifepristone.

◆ **Aspirin** is avoided in:
   ❖ children <16 (implicated in Reye's syndrome).
   ❖ patients with gout
   ❖ people with glucose-6-phosphate dehydrogenase deficiency.

◆ Porphyria attacks may be precipated by diclofenac.

Interactions

◆ Adverse effects of NSAIDs may be accentuated:
   ❖ **Bleeding** is increased by vasodilators (e.g. calcium channel blockers, nitrates, alcohol), anticoagulants and some herbal remedies, such as feverfew, *Ginkgo biloboa*, Siberian ginseng. Intravenous diclofenac should not be co-administered with any heparins. Long-term paracetamol enhances the actions of warfarin.

❖ **Gastrointestinal side effects** are increased by co-administration of more than one NSAID, alcohol, oral anticoagulants, corticosteroids or SSRIs.

❖ **Renal problems** are intensified by diuretics, ACE inhibitors, ciclosporin, vancomycin, tacrolimus.

◆ Anti-hypertensive effects of ACE inhibitors, calcium channel blockers, beta blockers and thiazide diuretics are reduced.

◆ Increased risk of hypoglycaemia with oral hypoglycaemics.

◆ NSAIDs may increase myoclonus associated with morphine.

◆ NSAIDs cause accumulation of: lithium, digoxin, quinolones, methotrexate. Aspirin does not interact with lithium, digoxin.

◆ Absorption of NSAIDs is increased by: metoclopramide and reduced by: cholestyramine, opioids, atropine, antipsychotics or tricyclic antidepressants. The effectiveness of aspirin may change if the pH of urine alters (e.g. due to antacid ingestion).

◆ Other drugs interacting with NSAIDs include: sodium valproate, phenytoin, thyroxine, moclobemide, zidovudine, ritonavir, baclofen, oral hypoglycaemics, and some antibiotics (ceftriaxone, chloramphenicol, sulphonamides, rifampicin, quinolones).

 # Paracetamol

Paracetamol is usually the analgesic of first choice, as it may offer adequate pain relief and is associated with fewer side effects. It may be combined with a low dose NSAID.

The main problem with paracetamol is risk of liver, kidney or pancreas damage in overdose, or even when the dose is only some 2–3 times that recommended. There are some reports of toxicity with long-term use at high prescribed doses. A few patients over-using alcohol and taking paracetamol within the prescribed range (below 4g/day) have developed liver failure.

Dose restrictions are advised in:

◆ children.

◆ frail elderly people.

◆ people with liver or kidney disease.

◆ those who over-use alcohol and go without food.

◆ patients who are HIV positive.

◆ patients taking other drugs which affect the liver e.g. tricyclic antidepressants, anti-epileptics, rifampicin, isoniazid, barbiturates.

Where metoclopramide is co-prescribed, absorption of paracetamol is increased, so lower doses may be appropriate.

21 Idiosyncratic drug reactions

This chapter considers some adverse drug reactions that can occur as idiosyncratic or hypersensitivity responses to many different drugs. These serious adverse events are rare, but emergency drugs and protocols are kept in place, should the need arise. Some individuals may be genetically susceptible to these problems.

Hypersensitivity or allergic responses

Hypersensitivity or allergic responses are possible with almost any drug, although antibiotics are particular offenders. These responses can also occur in association with insect stings or certain foods, such as eggs, fish or nuts. Individuals with a history of atopic disorders, such as asthma or eczema, are particularly vulnerable. Occasionally, the excipients (packing chemicals) used in tablets or injections or topical applications may be responsible for hypersensitivity responses. For example, zinc or other components of insulin injections may be responsible for rashes at injection sites. Polyoxyl castor oil (contained in ciclosporin and tacrolimus infusions) has been associated with anaphylactic reactions. Benzyl alcohol (contained in diclofenac and interferon alfa injections) has caused severe reactions in premature babies (BNF 2007).

Most drugs or their metabolites can combine with carrier proteins in the circulation to form **immunogens,** substances which produce an immune response. This may affect any one of several organs, such as skin, liver or bone marrow (Table 21.1). The severity of the hypersensitivity response is also variable, ranging from a temporary skin rash to life-threatening aplastic anaemia. A mild drug reaction usually takes the form of a red, erythematous rash or an urticarial ('nettle') rash (sometimes called hives). If at all possible, the offending drug is discontinued. For very serious infections, therapy may need to be continued, under careful observation. If the rash does not disappear, antihistamines or corticosteroids may be prescribed (Petri 2006). Once someone has experienced even a mild allergic skin reaction to a drug they are likely to be sensitised and are at increased risk of a more severe reaction, including anaphylaxis, at the next administration. However, the absolute risk may be relatively low, and prescribing will be dictated by clinical need, with increased vigilance (Aronson 2006, Petri 2006). **Patients are always asked if they have ever had an allergic response to any drug that is to be administered for the first time, and all allergies are documented.**

However, allergic reactions may appear when a drug is administered for the first time, presumably due to environmental exposures, for example, to penicillins (Petri 2006). Occupational exposure has, rarely, led to serious hypersensitivity reactions with betalactam antibiotics (Aronson 2006).

Allergic or hypersensitivity responses have been divided into 4 categories (Table 21.1). These involve different types of white cells and antibodies, and arise within different time frames. Some reactions may be delayed, or appear after the drug has been discontinued.

Table 21.1 Hypersensitivity responses: some examples

	Biological mechanism	Target organs	Clinical effects	Drugs (examples only)	Timing
Type I	Anaphylaxis Histamine release, causing inflammation and dilatation of blood vessels (see below)	Skin	Hives (urticaria), itching, rash, tissue swelling	Nearly all drugs, particularly when administered rapidly into a vein. Blood products. Vaccines (rarely).	Rapid onset (seconds to hours)
		Respiratory tract	Tightness of throat, sneezing, wheezing, shortness of breath, obstruction of airway. Immediate response in asthma		
		Blood vessels dilate, causing BP to fall	Hypotension, chest pain, irregular heart rate, feeling faint, 'aura'		
		Gut	Nausea, vomiting, abdominal cramps, diarrhoea		
Type II	Reactions against cells in the blood stream	Platelet concentration falls (thrombocytopenia) (Aster & Bougie 2007)	Bleeding, bruising and purpura	Quinine and similar drugs (cranberry juice contains quinine), linezolid, vancomycin, valproate	Subsides within months
		Red cells are split open	Haemolytic anaemia	Methyldopa, penicillins	
		White cell count falls, agranulocytosis (below), neutropenia	Infections, sore throat, fever	Sulfonamides, antipsychotics, some antiepileptics	
Type III	Inflammation due to release of destructive enzymes, known as 'serum sickness'	Skin, joints, kidneys	Hives, joint pains, swollen lymph glands, fever, kidney damage (below)	Antibiotics, lamotrigine, other anti-epileptics, iodides, gold salts, penicillamine	Subsides within days to weeks
		Respiratory system	Delayed asthma	Some antidepressants, e.g. fluoxetine, amphetamines	
		Vasculitis: damage to blood vessels and impaired oxygen delivery to tissues, usually lower legs	Painful ulceration and necrosis Often preceded by itching	Penicillins, ACE inhibitors	
Type IV	Delayed cell-mediated immune response. More common in those who are HIV positive.	Skin	Oedema and rash Contact dermatitis	Handling penicillins, phenothiazines, opioids Topical anti-histamines, local anaesthetics*	Prolonged exposure
		Skin: toxic epidermal necrolysis	Widespread loss of skin, leaving red, scalded areas	Antibiotics, ACE inhibitors, lamotrigine	
		Liver	Liver damage (below)	Anti-epileptics	
		Inflammation of mucous membranes, the Stevens–Johnson syndrome, affects all lining tissues of the body.	Swelling of mucous membranes of mouth and eyes, rash, damage to heart, central nervous system changes, joint pains	Antibiotics	

It is not always possible to assign an allergic reaction to a specific mechanism, and authorities may differ in their classification of individual reactions (Klaassen 2001, Shear 2007).
* When handling drugs which can cause contact dermatitis, practitioners are advised to wear gloves (Smith et al. 2008).

Many patients who report that they are 'allergic to penicillin' do not demonstrate hypersensitivity responses, and can be administered penicillin safely. However, without testing, there is no way of identifying such patients. Therefore, if penicillin is needed and the diagnosis of drug allergy is in doubt, skin prick tests may be undertaken. Skin prick tests involve administration of a very small dose of the allergen. Therefore, they are undertaken in hospitals where emergency facilities are available, as they can, very occasionally, trigger anaphylaxis. However, these only detect type 1 hypersensitivity responses. If the skin prick tests are negative (no reaction seen), it is usually considered safe to administer penicillin (Solensky et al. 2002). Not everyone with positive skin prick tests will develop clinical allergy: only some two thirds of those with positive skin tests and history of allergy will develop symptoms on re-administration of penicillin (Stern et al. 2001), but practitioners consider these risks too great.

Anaphylaxis and angioedema

The most immediate type of hypersensitivity response is anaphylaxis. This can also arise from allergens in food, latex, insect stings or following exercise. It is estimated that 1–15% of the population are at risk (Neugut et al. 2001), and about 1 in 2,000 injections of betalactam antibiotics is followed by anaphylaxis (Aronson 2006). Some of this variation has arisen as a result of inconsistency in diagnosing and reporting of anaphylaxis (Sampson et al. 2005). It is important that anaphylaxis is promptly recognised, as delay in treatment may have serious consequences, or prove fatal.

Anaphylaxis occurs within minutes or hours of administration of the allergen, and within seconds to an hour after injection. Therefore, patients are observed for at least 15 minutes after the first dose of a new intravenous drug. Anaphylaxis is characterised by: sudden onset of urticarial rash (hives); flushing, tissue swelling (particularly around the mouth); obstruction of the respiratory tract, bronchoconstriction (narrowing of airways); and/or hypotension; diarrhoea, sometimes. Bronchospasm, causing sudden and worsening difficulty in breathing may be the first indication of a problem. Dilatation of blood vessels may cause hypotension, which may be followed by circulatory collapse and incontinence. The patient may visibly swell and lose consciousness as blood pressure plummets. Other presentations are possible. Death is most likely to occur from oedema obstructing the airways (angioedema) (Sampson et al. 2006).

Almost any medication can cause a hypersensitivity response; common offenders include:

◆ anti-microbials and antibiotics.
◆ hormone preparations.
◆ dextrans.
◆ heparin.
◆ vaccines.
◆ blood products.
◆ iron injections.
◆ local anaesthetics.
◆ streptokinase.

Where drugs have similar chemical structures, **some cross allergies exist**, for example some (10% of) people who are allergic to penicillins will also be allergic to cephalosporins.

Management of anaphylaxis is described in the current edition of the BNF. This involves stopping the drug, assessing the situation, calling for help, maintaining the airway, positioning the patient, administering oxygen and adrenaline, monitoring vital signs and preparing fluid resuscitation. Adrenaline is usually given intra-muscularly into the lateral thigh (Figure 21.1). Lower doses are prescribed for self-administration, for example as Epipen®, to those who develop anaphylaxis to insect stings or foods.

In extreme emergencies, if the circulation is inadequate, adrenaline may be given by slow intravenous injection (Sampson *et al.* 2006). **Two different strengths of adrenaline/ epinephrine solution are available. This could lead to confusion in an emergency: should the stronger (1 in 1,000) solution be administered intravenously, fatalities could occur.**

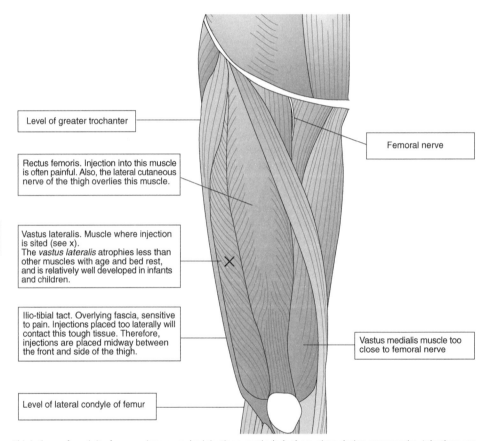

Level of greater trochanter

Femoral nerve

Rectus femoris. Injection into this muscle is often painful. Also, the lateral cutaneous nerve of the thigh overlies this muscle.

Vastus lateralis. Muscle where injection is sited (see x).
The *vastus lateralis* atrophies less than other muscles with age and bed rest, and is relatively well developed in infants and children.

Ilio-tibial tact. Overlying fascia, sensitive to pain. Injections placed too laterally will contact this tough tissue. Therefore, injections are placed midway between the front and side of the thigh.

Vastus medialis muscle too close to femoral nerve

Level of lateral condyle of femur

This is the preferred site for many intramuscular injections, particularly those given during emergencies. Injections are placed in the central third of the thigh, a hand's breadth above the knee (lateral condyle of femur) and a hand's breadth below the greater trochanter of the femur. There are few nerves and blood vessels at this site.

Z track technique is used, Fig. 10.3.

The thigh contains the bulkiest muscles of the body. The vastus lateralis in the lateral aspect of the anterior thigh is relatively distant from major nerves and blood vessels, but has been associated with femoral nerve injury. It is able to accommodate up to 5ml. of injection in an adult (1.0ml. in children under 3 and 2.5ml. in those under 15) (Hayes *et al.* 2003). However, patients report more pain from injections administered into the thigh than the buttock (McKenry and Salerno 2003), and any scars and nodules are immediately visible to the patient

In the front of the thigh, the medial aspect of the vastus medialis is close to the femoral artery, femoral vein and saphenous nerve, and this is not usually recommended for intramuscular injections.

Figure 21.1 Intramuscular injection site in the anterolateral thigh

Adrenaline can have adverse effects. It is only administered to seriously ill patients, with extreme caution and close monitoring of vital signs and ECG. Practitioners monitor for:

◆ cardiac dysrhythmia.

◆ sudden rise in BP, which could cause cerebral haemorrhage.

◆ vomiting (and subsequent choking).

◆ pulmonary oedema.

◆ hyperglycaemia.

Adrenaline may not be effective in patients taking beta blockers (such as atenolol, labetolol) and intravenous salbutamol or glucagon may be needed (Sampson et al. 2006). Due to beta blockade, there may be no response from beta receptors, and no relief of obstructed airways. Beta blockade allows adrenaline to act on only the alpha receptors, causing a sudden, severe rise in BP and bradycardia. Extra care may also be needed for patients prescribed drugs which block alpha receptors (such as clonidine for pain or hypertension) (Baxter 2006). In theory, other drugs which block alpha receptors, such as antipsychotics, tricyclic antidepressants or drugs for prostatic hypertrophy, could cause similar problems (glossary, adrenergic receptors).

Intravenous antihistamine (chlorphenamine/chlorpheniramine) is also administered and continued for 24–48 hours to prevent relapse, together with close observation (BNF 2007). It is estimated that 10% of patients with anaphylaxis will not respond to treatment (Sampson et al. 2005).

A few drugs, such as vancomycin, opioids, can cause histamine release. This is associated with severe flushing and hypotension. This reaction may be confused with anaphylaxis, but requires different management (Aronson 2006).

179

Drug induced bone marrow damage/suppression

The red bone marrow contains stem cells which give rise to:

◆ white blood cells, which form the immune system and prevent infection.

◆ red blood cells, which transport oxygen and carbon dioxide.

◆ platelets, which are important in blood clotting.

These are continuously being broken down and need to be renewed. In the non-pregnant state, cells of the bone marrow are among the most actively dividing in the body. Therefore, they are affected when DNA formation is hindered by anticancer drugs or lack of folic acid or vitamin B_{12}. Rarely, the bone marrow is damaged in idiosyncratic adverse drug reactions associated with some antipsychotics, antiepileptics, antibiotics, antidepressants, diuretics, ACE inhibitors, anti-emetics, anti-diabetic agents and anti-thyroid drugs.

There are several types of white cells. The most numerous are the neutrophils, which represent the body's first line of defence against invading micro-organisms and infection. If the bone marrow is damaged, these are no longer formed and there is a risk of severe and overwhelming infection. If a patient develops a low white cell count as a result of drug exposure, it is essential that this is recognised promptly, as the patient can be treated with colony stimulating factors (such as filgrastim) in intensive care.

The white cells of patients prescribed clozapine are monitored by regular monthly blood tests, and more frequently on initiation of therapy. However, for other drugs, diagnosis relies on clinicians recognising the signs of rapidly-developing infection, particularly sore throat and fever, and arranging urgent full blood counts. To minimise risk:

◆ Ask patients to report infections, e.g. sore throat, fever, weakness as these may indicate serious adverse reactions.

◆ Obtain full blood count to evaluate these symptoms.

◆ Obtain regular full blood counts in patients with collagen vascular diseases, such as systemic lupus.

A low white blood cell count may indicate:

◆ bone marrow disease.

◆ damage from radiotherapy.

◆ nutritional deficiency.

◆ immuno-compromised state, such as HIV infection or immunosuppressant drugs

◆ drug-induced damage (rarely).

Changes in white cell numbers should always be reported promptly.

Drug-induced liver damage

The liver can be damaged by a wide range of drugs and herbal remedies. Damage may be dose-related, for example paracetamol, alcohol, allopurinol, azathiaprine. For other drugs, e.g. anti-epileptics, erythromycin, the relationship to dose is less clear. These rare adverse effects may be idiosyncratic allergic responses. Liver damage may be acute or take months to accumulate.

Everything that is eaten, including orally administered drugs, passes from the gut into the liver, where it is metabolised and detoxified by liver enzymes. Therefore, the liver is vulnerable to damage by toxins or metabolites, particularly when high doses are administered. Not everyone has the correct balance of enzymes needed to metabolise some drugs safely. In some cases, harmful, rather than safe, metabolites are produced, and these damage liver cells; these problems are not dose-related, and are not predictable (examples include the antitubercular drug isoniazid, NSAIDs). There are no tests to assess the liver's ability/capacity to metabolise and eliminate medication (Perucca *et al.* 2006).

It is difficult to recognise and diagnose liver damage from clinical history and examination alone: persistent nausea, fullness in the upper abdomen, abdominal pain or confusion are possible early signs. Jaundice usually occurs late in the course of the illness, when the concentration of bilirubin is three times above the normal limit. Therefore, for some drugs, e.g. valproate, carbamazepine, regular liver function tests are recommended to detect any liver damage at an early stage, so that the drug can be withdrawn before damage reaches a critical threshold, and while the liver is still able to recover.

Tests to assess liver damage

If liver cells are damaged, their enzymes leak out into the circulation, where they can be measured in liver function tests (LFTs) on venous blood samples. The enzymes include alanine amino transferase and aspartate amino transferase (ALT and AST), which are important in protein synthesis and only occur in liver cells. Raised concentrations of AST and ALT indicate that liver cells have recently been damaged, and their contents are passing into the circulation. This occurs in all forms of liver injury, including infectious hepatitis. **The rise in liver enzyme concentrations may only be transient, and have no serious consequences, but prescribers should always be informed.** However, liver function tests only detect ongoing damage. If liver damage has occurred previously, leaving only scar tissue, there are no enzymes to leak into the circulation, and concentrations of AST and ALT will be normal.

An indication of such damage (known as cirrhosis) can often be estimated from a detailed history of alcohol intake.

Some drugs (e.g. chlorpromazine, oestrogens) or their metabolites occasionally damage the small bile ducts, gradually causing them to block, and impeding the passage of bile into the gut (known as cholestasis). When this occurs, the enzyme alkaline phosphatase passes from the bile ducts into the circulation, and can be measured in venous blood samples. Without bile, fats cannot be absorbed, remain in the gut and pass into the faeces. Fatty, light coloured, malodorous stools may be the first sign of malabsorption, caused by liver failure, and should be reported. Another example of long-term liver damage is the deposition of fat in liver cells caused by steroids, valproate or tetracyclines.

It is not always possible to identify a cause for liver damage. Attributing liver damage to a drug may depend on clinical judgement as to timing of exposure and the presence of other risk factors, such as alcohol use (Lee & Senior 2005). With age, the liver becomes more vulnerable to drug-induced injury (Ginsberg *et al.* 2005).

If liver function is impaired, for any reason, the body's ability to eliminate most drugs is impaired. Some drugs are given in reduced doses e.g. paracetamol, whereas others are avoided altogether e.g. oestrogens. (Appendix 2 of the BNF gives detailed information.)

Drug-induced kidney damage

Many drugs can damage the kidney, including NSAIDs, ACE inhibitors, gentamicin, lithium. Some drugs (e.g. thiazide diuretics, cocaine), may damage the filtration mechanism (the glomeruli, see Figure 3.1) either directly, or in relation to a hypersensitivity response (Table 21.1). Others can affect the kidney tubules, particularly at higher doses e.g. gentamicin, cisplatin (for cancer) and ciclosporin (an immunosuppressant). A few drugs (e.g. statins) can (rarely) cause muscle breakdown (rhabdomyolysis); this releases muscle breakdown products (myoglobin) which affect the flow of urine in the tubules, causing blockage and necrosis. A further cause of kidney damage is the deposition of crystals in the renal tubules by sulfadiazine (in co-trimoxazole, Septrin®), acyclovir or indavir. These drugs are most likely to be prescribed for patients with HIV infection, who are often dehydrated. The deposition of crystals is less likely if the flow of urine is high, therefore, patients prescribed these drugs need careful fluid balance monitoring to ensure good hydration (Markowitz & Perazella 2005). Renal damage may be followed by scarring, which reduces future renal function. Patients should be informed that smoking intensifies any renal damage.

Most (about two-thirds) drugs are eliminated *via* the kidneys. If drugs damage the kidney, the kidney loses its ability to eliminate the offending drug, and a vicious circle, leading to drug accumulation and further kidney damage, develops.

Renal function must be monitored in patients prescribed drugs which damage the kidney, so that the drug can be withdrawn before too much renal tissue is lost, and the patient develops signs and symptoms of kidney failure. In the most serious cases, kidney damage results in the patient needing life-long dialysis.

Tests of kidney function

If kidney function is impaired, drugs may be given in reduced doses e.g. valproate, and others may be avoided altogether e.g. tetracyclines, lithium, metformin. (Appendix 3 of the BNF gives detailed information.) Kidney function is tested to ensure that medications will not accumulate in the body and assess any drug-induced kidney damage.

Serum creatinine

One of the kidney's most important functions is excretion of potentially harmful nitrogenous waste, such as urea and creatinine. Measuring these in venous blood samples gives an indication of the health of the kidney. However, this needs careful interpretation.

Creatinine concentration is conveniently measured from venous blood samples (normal range 62–124 micromol/l, varying slightly between laboratories). Creatinine concentration rises above normal when 50% of nephrons have been damaged. Values >700 micromol/l, indicate severe renal compromise. If patients are reviewed regularly, serial measurements of serum creatinine are sufficient to highlight any changes in kidney function, provided patients maintain relatively constant body mass and dietary intake (Rodrigo et al., 2002).

The prescriber should be informed if a patient's serum creatinine concentration increases, as drug doses will normally need to be reduced, and the prescriber may wish to order further investigations of kidney function.

Patients vulnerable to renal damage e.g. those with repeated UTI, diabetes or cardiovascular disease, older people and those prescribed certain drugs e.g. lithium, NSAIDs, ACE inhibitors, ciclosporin, tacrolimus, aminosalicylates, metformin should have serum creatinine concentration monitored regularly.

Creatinine is derived from creatine, which is made in the liver from amino acids. Creatine is an energy store in skeletal muscle. It is metabolised to creatinine and excreted into the plasma at a fairly constant rate. Serum creatinine concentration depends on the balance between production by muscle and elimination by kidneys.

The amount of creatinine in the circulation depends on both the muscle mass and the renal function of the individual. Someone who is immobile or with very little muscle e.g. an older female, will have a low creatinine concentration: for older bedbound women with normal renal function this is approximately 40–70 micromol/l. Therefore, when kidney function is impaired in such patients, any rise in serum creatinine concentration will still give a test result within the 'normal' range. Therefore, basing an initial assessment of kidney function solely on serum creatinine concentration can be misleading, and may not give an accurate assessment of the kidney's ability to eliminate drugs (Skorecki et al. 2001). Other measures of kidney function are often needed.

GFR (glomerular filtration rate)

GFR is considered the best overall measure of the kidneys' ability to eliminate drugs in health and disease (Levey et al. 1999). It is the volume of fluid filtered into the nephrons every minute, i.e. the sum of the volume of filtrate formed in all the functioning nephrons in the kidneys each minute. The normal GFR for a standard male (of body surface area $1.73m^2$) is 100ml/min.; the value for a female is 90% of this. A GFR below 60ml/min./$1.73m^2$ surface area indicates renal disorder, and is associated with increased risk of cardiovascular disease (Stevens and Levey 2005).

An estimate of the GFR (the eGFR) is obtained from laboratory reports. The eGFR is calculated from venous blood samples analysed for serum concentrations of creatinine, taking age, gender and ethnicity into account. Age and gender are always shown on 'patient stickers'. eGFR gives the GFR adjusted for a person of standard body surface area ($1.73m^2$). An eGFR >90ml/min./$1.73m^2$ indicates good kidney function. If eGFR is below 60ml/min./$1.73m^2$, the doctor should be informed (Joint Specialty Committee on Renal Medicine (JSC) 2006).

It is sometimes necessary to know the absolute or unadjusted GFR for calculating drug doses, and other measures can be used (Levey et al. 1999).

GFR (and therefore urine output and drug elimination) are affected by:

◆ changes in blood flow to the kidneys e.g dehydration (including the use of diuretics), shock, heart failure, administration of NSAIDs or ACEIs.

◆ renal disorders and loss of nephrons (e.g. repeated UTI, pre-eclampsia, long-term prostatic enlargement).

◆ life cycle (below).

In acute care, monitoring of urine output and specific gravity is important. If people are acutely ill, blood flow and renal function can change rapidly, affecting drug concentrations. If the volume of urine is too low, the kidneys are at risk of damage. Urine output <0.5ml/kg/hour indicates that the circulation is seriously compromised and renal blood supply and oxygen delivery are inadequate (Jevon & Ewens 2002). Urine output measurement less than 30ml/hr should be reported to the doctor managing the patient, because renal damage may be occurring, and drugs may rapidly accumulate, and reach toxic concentrations (Berman *et al.* 2008).

Serum potassium

The kidneys are responsible for maintaining potassium balance: as renal failure develops, potassium may accumulate and cause cardiac problems. A potassium concentration above the normal range for the reporting laboratory (typically >5.1 mmol/.) should be reported to prescriber. If concentration of potassium is >6.0 mmol/l, the prescriber will usually change medication, for example withdraw NSAIDs (JSE 2006).

Urine specific gravity

The kidneys control the body's salt and water balance (Figure 3.1). They filter 180 litres of water each day, but only 1–2 litres are passed as urine. The kidney tubules adjust the amount of water and salt eliminated so that the osmotic pressure (or salt and water balance) of the body remains constant. This is monitored by assessing fluid balance and testing the concentrating ability of the kidney tubules. Health of, or damage to, renal tubules is assessed by testing the specific gravity (or density) of urine, which reflects the concentrating ability of the tubules.

Urine composition

The kidneys filter the blood, so that cells and large molecules (mainly proteins) are retained in the circulation as urine is formed. Filtration takes place in the glomeruli, through the pores in the glomerular basement membrane. This is damaged in certain diseases e.g. diabetes, systemic lupus, infections, or by environmental toxins e.g. lead, mercury, and some drugs e.g. gold salts, NSAIDs, ACEIs. If the glomerular basement membrane is diseased or damaged, its pores enlarge (holes appear) and proteins (micro-albumins, then albumins) leak out and appear in the urine, where they can be measured. **Early damage to the glomerular basement membrane can be detected by the presence of protein in the urine.** This is assessed by measuring the protein/creatinine ratio in the urine; a value above 45mg/mmol indicates renal damage. This is equivalent to a concentration of protein >150mg/day in 24-hour urine collection (Redmond & McCelland 2006). However, 24-hour urine collection is impractical in primary care, and not advised (JSC 2006).

Urine can be tested for protein, using dipstick reagents, preferably when the patient has not been exercising. (However, these can be contaminated by vaginal discharge or menstrual flow.) If a positive result is obtained, an early morning urine sample should be sent for laboratory analysis of the protein/creatinine ratio and a mid-stream urine sample should be sent for investigation of possible infection (JSC 2006).

Fluid balance

Change in the volume of urine, which manifests itself as incontinence or nocturia could be the first indication of renal impairment, and may warrant further investigation. **Deterioration in continence may indicate declining renal function. Direct inquiries should be made and kidney function should be tested.** (See Box 21.1.)

Box 21.1 Summary of renal function tests

Venous blood sample for measurement of the concentration of:
    creatinine
    urea
    potassium

Urine samples for:
    specific gravity
    detection of infection
    concentration of albumin and microalbumin
    protein/creatinine ratio

Fluid balance:
    An estimate of daily intake should be possible in all care settings.

Continence assessment.

Change in kidney function during the life cycle

Neonates

The GFR of neonates is 30–40% of adult values. Therefore, there is a danger that certain drugs may accumulate following neonatal or maternal administration (e.g. magnesium) or during breastfeeding (e.g. lithium).

Children

By the age of 12, drug elimination reaches adult values. With the exception of certain drugs acting on the CNS (such as SSRIs), adult doses are appropriate for those aged >12 years (BNF 2007). Children's doses are sometimes quoted as per kg body weight. However, for obese children ideal, rather than actual, body weight is often a better basis for this calculation, and adult doses should not be exceeded (Ginsberg et al. 2002).

Pregnancy

In pregnancy GFR increases 30–50%, in keeping with increased metabolic demands. This increases the elimination of certain drugs, and women prescribed anti-epileptics should be monitored closely. The increase in GFR reduces serum creatinine concentration. 'Normal' laboratory values change during pregnancy. Any serum creatinine value over 70 micromol/l (80 micromol/l in the last week of pregnancy) is indicative of possible renal compromise and need for further investigations (Perrone et al. 1992, Milman et al. 2007).

Older adults

After about 60, most individuals' ability to eliminate drugs declines: by age 80, clearance has declined by 50% (Ginsberg *et al.* 2005). Therefore, older patients are prescribed lower doses of most drugs. The body has a substantial reserve of renal function. Renal function and reserve decline with age in about two thirds of people (Perucca *et al.* 2006). Often, this will produce no signs and symptoms, unless drugs are taken which require renal elimination.

◆ With long-term therapy, as renal function declines with age, drugs may accumulate and adverse effects may appear gradually or suddenly e.g. digoxin, sedatives. Sometimes an acute episode of dehydration (for example due to fever) is superimposed on gradually declining renal function, and adverse effects may appear for the first time, although the patient may have been taking the drug for several years. Therefore, extra monitoring is required when patients develop a fever, reduce their fluid intake or commence diuretic therapy.

◆ With long-term drug therapy, regular assessment of renal function is essential. Increasing serum creatinine concentration or rising GFR should be reported:

  ❖ Fluid intake should be explored.

  ❖ Strategies to reduce risk of cardiovascular disease should be reviewed. (Raised serum creatinine indicates increased risk of cardiovascular events.)

  ❖ The prescriber may need to revise the choice or dose of medication.

Gender

Women have a lower GFR than men. For example, women eliminate 5FU (a cytotoxic drug) more slowly than men, and, without appropriate dose reductions, experience increased toxicity (Hurria & Lichtman 2007). The combined effect of age and gender means that older women have reduced ability to eliminate drugs, and an increased risk of adverse effects.

For full lists of drug-induced conditions see Kelly (2000) and Wood (2001).

Glossary

Acetylcholine	Neurotransmitter of the parasympathetic nervous system
Adrenergic receptors of the sympathetic nervous system (SNS)	These respond to adrenaline and noradrenaline. They are classified: 1. **Alpha receptors** ◆ Alpha$_1$ receptors regulate vasoconstriction, blood flow and BP, smooth muscle and sphincters of the gut and urethra, and the size of the pupil ◆ Alpha$_2$ receptors regulate noradrenaline/norepinephrine secretion 2. **Beta receptors** ◆ Beta$_1$ receptors regulate the heart ◆ Beta$_2$ receptors regulate the airways, the liver, the renin-angiotensin mechanism, blood vessels. Adrenaline/epinephrine acts preferentially on beta$_2$ receptors ◆ Beta$_3$ receptors regulate energy production in brown fat
Agonist	A substance having a specific cellular affinity that produces a predictable response; also, a chemical capable of stimulating a cell receptor
Agranulocytosis	A marked reduction in the number of circulating granular leukocytes, particularly neutrophils. This renders the patient very liable to serious infections. Unrecognised and untreated, these overwhelming infections can be fatal
Akathisia	Motor restlessness with sensation of quivering and wanting to move about constantly. This is usually caused by drugs that affect areas of the brain controlling posture and movement
Anaphylactic reaction	A serious life-threatening hypersensitivity reaction, characterised by low blood pressure, shock and difficulty in breathing
Antagonist	A chemical that can occupy a cell receptor without stimulating it and thereby block the action of agonists for that receptor
Antibiotics	Natural substances that inhibit the growth of, or kill, bacteria. Sometimes widened to substances that inhibit all micro-organisms
Anti-microbials	Substances which suppress the growth of micro-organisms
Bioavailability	A measure of absorption or the fractional extent to which the drug dose reaches its site of action (Wilkinson 2001 p. 5)
Bioequivalent	Products are bioequivalent if their rates and extents of bioavailability of their active ingredient are not significantly different under suitable test conditions (Wilkinson 2001 p. 8)

Bisphosphonates	Drugs e.g. alendronic acid, disodium etidronate, prescribed for osteoporosis, bone pain and Paget's disease
Cell cycle	Dividing cells go through phases: forming components of DNA; forming DNA; preparing for cell division; cell division. After division, some cells leave the cycle and enter a 'resting phase', which can last for several years
Cholinergic	Relating to acetylcholine, a neurotransmitter in the central nervous system and parasympathetic nervous system
Diuresis	Increased excretion of urine
Dose related or dose dependent	There is often wide individual variation in the changes in body function brought about by drugs, and doses are adjusted to individual needs. However, there is usually a relationship between drug dose and patient response, that is, the higher the dose, the greater the effect on the body. Dose-related adverse effects are more likely to occur at higher doses. For example, the risk of bleeding increases as the dose of anti-coagulant increases
Enteral	By way of the gastrointestinal tract
Enteric coated preparation	A special coating applied to tablets or capsules which prevents release and absorption of their contents until they reach the intestine
Enzyme	Protein-based catalyst that accelerates the body's chemical reactions
Excipient	A vehicle added to a prescription to confer a suitable consistency or form to a pharmaceutical product
Fibroblasts	Cells found in connective tissues which produce collagen and elastin fibres and are responsible for healing
Haematocrit	The **haematocrit** value (as seen on full blood count forms) is the percentage of whole blood occupied by cells. Normal values are $47 \pm 7\%$ for men, $42 \pm 5\%$ for women and children. Raised values are associated with dehydration. Haematocrit is a crucial measure of blood viscosity (stickiness) and, therefore, the risk of clotting (Guyton & Hall 2000)
Half-life	The elimination half-life for each drug is the time taken for the concentration of the drug in plasma and the amount of drug in the body to fall to half its maximum value (Buxton 2006 p.16). Duration of action increases in direct proportion to half-life. With repeated dosing, many drugs accumulate until they reach a plateau or steady state. The time taken for this is between 3–5 times the drug's elimination half-life (Endrenyi 2007). The full effects of the drug and dose-related side effects (Chapter 1) often do not appear until the steady state is reached. If the half-life of the drug is known, it is possible to predict when dose-related adverse effects are most likely to appear for the first time

Heart block	Heart block slows the heart rate and reduces the heart's output. This can impair oxygen delivery to the brain, and cause the patient to collapse. It is diagnosed on the ECG if the PR interval is greater than 200ms or 5 small squares. PR interval = start of P to start of Q
Hypokalaemia	Serum potassium concentration below normal values. These are 3.5–5.1 mmol/l. Hypokalaemia may cause a range of problems from vague symptoms of weakness, constipation, depression to sudden cardiac events
Hyponatraemia	Serum sodium ion concentration below normal values. These are 135–145 mmol/l. Headache, lethargy, anorexia, nausea and vomiting may be early signs of hyponatraemia. Serious symptoms develop if serum sodium concentration falls below 120 mmol/l.
International normalised ratio (INR)	The ratio of the prothrombin time of the patient's blood sample to the prothrombin time of a standard blood sample. The prothrombin time is a measure of the time taken for clot formation when a tissue thromboplastin reagent is added. It effectively measures the activity of prothrombin, fibrinogen and factors V, VII & X
Jejunum	The portion of the small intestine that extends from the duodenum to the ileum
Ketogenic diet	A high fat, low carbohydrate and normal protein diet causing ketosis
Lactose intolerance	Some 70% non-Caucasian adults lack the enzyme lactase in the GI tract. Therefore, lactose in milk and similar sugars in lactulose cannot be broken down, and remain in the gut. The undigested, unabsorbed lactose passes to the large intestine, where it is fermented by bacteria, producing acidic stools and flatulence. Therefore, milk, dairy products or lactulose can cause abdominal pain and distension and urgent diarrhoea
Macrophage	Macrophages are phagocytic: they can engulf any foreign material, such as bacteria, viruses, dust particles, worn-out, dead or abnormal body cells. In this way, they act as a general 'rubbish collection and disposal' system
MAOI	Monoamine oxidase inhibitors, drugs that interfere with the action of monoamine oxidase. These drugs slow the breakdown of certain neurotransmitters, such as norepinephrine and related chemicals, such as tyramine. They are prescribed for the management of depressive illness
Myoclonus	Myoclonus is repetitive involuntary muscle contraction, jerking or shaking due to imbalance in the normal controls of skeletal muscle tension. It may be distressing to both patients and carers
Neurotransmitter	Chemical messengers passing from one neurone to the next, across the synaptic cleft. This is a space of about 20 nanometers

	between adjacent neurones. Examples include, acetylcholine, histamine, adrenaline/epinephrine, noradrenaline/norepinephrine, dopamine, serotonin
Nystagmus	Involuntary rapid movements of the eyeballs. Movements may be horizontal, vertical or rotatary. Indication of brain stem, vestibular and cerebellar disturbance
Opioids	Any preparation acting on the body's opioid receptors, e.g. morphine, diamorphine, codeine, naloxone
Phaeochromocytoma	A tumour derived from the cells of the adrenal medulla, secreting adrenaline and/or noradrenaline
Porphyria	The porphyrias are a group of <u>rare</u> inherited conditions, in which enzymes needed to make haemoglobin are deficient or absent. Therefore, intermediate compounds accumulate, and can cause neurological disturbance, psychosis, abdominal pain, skin changes or urine pigmentation. In susceptible, but asymptomatic, people, this condition can be triggered by administration of certain medications (see Introduction)
QT interval prolongation	This is diagnosed if QT interval is more than 456ms or 11 small squares. QT interval = start of Q to end of T. It indicates a high risk of a cardiac event
Rhabdomyolosis	The destruction of skeletal muscle cells
Serotonin syndrome	A rare, but dangerous, complication of therapy with SSRIs. The increased serotonin concentration in the central nervous system may cause hyperthermia together with mental state changes and, sometimes, cardiovascular or movement problems
Shock	Inadequate delivery of oxygen to the tissues, due to acute failure of the peripheral circulation. Causes include: excessive fluid loss, such as haemorrhage; acute cardiac failure; sepsis; and adrenal failure
Teratogenesis	Impaired development of fetal organs, leading to structural or functional abnormalities (Koren *et al.* 1998 p.1128).
Teratogenic	Causing impaired development of fetal organs, leading to structural or functional abnormalities
Therapeutic range	Drug plasma concentrations which will provide therapy but avoid toxicity to the patient. Above the therapeutic range, toxic effects may appear. Below the therapeutic range, the drug does not have the desired effect
Tinnitus	A sensation of noises, such as ringing, buzzing, roaring in the ears, usually due to disturbance of the fluids of the inner ear
Toxicity	The quality of being poisonous

References

ABPI (Association of the British Pharmaceutical Industry) (2007) *Compendium of Data sheets and Summaries of Product Characteristics* (updated yearly). Datapharm Publications Ltd (Pharmacy Dept): London. emc.medicines.org.uk

Abraham, P., Avenell, A., Watson, W., Park, C., Bevan, J. (2003) Antithyroid drug regimen for treating Graves' hyperthyroidism. *Cochrane Database Systematic Review* 2003(4).

Adams, C., Rathbone, J., Thornley, *et al.* (2005) Chlorpromazine for schizophrenia: a Cochrane systematic review of 50 years of randomised controlled trials. *BioMed Central Medicine* 3(15). http://www.biomedcentral.com/1741–7015/3/15

ALLHAT Collaborative research group (2002) Major outcomes in high risk hypertensive patients randomized to antiotensin-converting enzyme inhibitor or calcium channel blocker vs. diuretic. *Journal of the American Medical Association* 288: 2981–97.

Aronson, J.K. (ed.) (2006) *Meyler's Side Effects of Drugs: The International Encyclopedia of Adverse Drug Reactions and Interactions*. Elsevier: New York. http://www.sciencedirect.com/science/referenceworks/0444510052

Aster, R., Bougie, D. (2007) Drug-induced immune thrombocytopenia. *New England Journal of Medicine* 357(6): 580–7.

Audit Commission (2001) *A Spoonful of Sugar: Medicines Management in NHS Hospitals.* Audit Commission: London.

Awad, A.G. (1999) Behavioural and subjective effects. In: Kane, J.M. (ed.) *Managing the Side Effects of Drug Therapy in Schizophrenia*. Science Press: London.

Balkau, B., Shipley, M., Jarrett, R.J. *et al.* (1998) High blood glucose concentration is a risk factor for mortality in middle-aged nondiabetic men. 20-year follow-up in the Whitehall Study, the Paris Prospective Study, and the Helsinki Policemen Study. *Diabetes Care* 21(3): 360–7.

Bandolier Extra (2003) *Evidence-based Healthcare: Acute Pain.* www. Ebandolier.com accessed Sept. 2007. http://www.jr2.ox.ac.uk/Bandolier/Extraforbando/APain.pdf

BAPEN (British Association for Parenteral and Enteral Nutrition) (2003) *Administering Drugs via Enteral Feeding Tubes: A Practical Guide*. BAPEN: London.

Barbui, C., Hotopf, M. (2001) Amitriptyline v. the rest: still the leading antidepressant after 40 years of randomised controlled trials. *British Journal of Psychiatry* 178: 129–44.

Barnes, T. (1989) A Rating scale for Drug-Induced Akathisia. *British Journal of Psychiatry* 154: 672–6.

Bartlett, N., Koczwara, B. (2002) Control of nausea and vomiting after chemotherapy: what is the evidence? *Internal Medicine Journal* 32: 401–7.

Barzo, B., Moretti, M., Mareels, G., van Tittelboom, T., Koren, G. (1999) Reporting bias in retrospective ascertainment of drug-induced embryopathy. *Lancet* 354: 1700–1.

Baxter, K. (2006) *Stockley's Drug Interactions*, 7th edition. Blackwell Science: Oxford.

Bennett, N. (1994) Hypertension in the elderly. *Lancet* 344: 447–9.

Berard, A., Ramos, E., Rey, E., Blais, L., St-Andre, M., Oraichi, D. (2007) First trimester exposure to paroxetine and risk of cardiac malformations in infants: the importance of dosage. Birth Defects Research Part B. *Developmental and Reproductive Toxicology* 80(1): 18–27.

Berg, D. (1999) *Advanced Clinical Skills*. Blackwell Science: Oxford.

Berman, A., Snyder, S., Kozier, B., Erb, G. (2008) *Kozier and Erb's Fundamentals of Nursing*, 8th edition. Pearson: Upper Saddle River, New Jersey.

British National Formulary (BNF) (2007) no. 53, British Medical Association and the Royal Pharmaceutical Society of Great Britain: London. bnf.org

British Thoracic Society (BTS) (2005) *British Guideline on the Management of Asthma*. BTS: London, also 2007 update on http: //www.brit-thoracic.org.uk.

Brown, M.J., Palmer, C.A., Castaigne, P., *et al.* (2000) Morbidity and mortality in patients randomised to double-blind treatment with a long-acting calcium-channel blocker or diuretic in the International Nifedipine GITS study: Intervention as a Goal in Hypertension Treatment (INSIGHT). *Lancet* 356: 366–72.

Budnitz, D., Pollock, D., Weidenbach, K., Mendelsohn, A., Schroeder, T., Annest, J. (2006) National surveillance of emergency department visits for outpatient adverse drug events. *Journal of the American Medical Association* 296(15): 1858–66.

Burr, R., Nuseibeh, I. (1997) Urinary catheter blockage depends on urine pH, calcium and rate of flow. *Spinal Cord* 35(8): 521–5.

Buxton, I. (2006) Pharmacokinetics and pharmacodynamics, pp.1–39. In: Brunton, L., Lazo, J., Parker, K. (eds) *Goodman & Gilman's: The Pharmacological Basis of Therapeutics*, 11th edition. McGraw-Hill: New York.

CARIS (2006) The CARIS review including 1998–2005 data. *NHS Wales*. www.wales.nhs.uk/caris

Carlson, C., Hornbuckle, K., DeLisle, F., Kryzhanovskaya, L., Breier, A., Cavazzoni, P. (2006) Diabetes mellitus and antipsychotic treatment in the United Kingdom. *European Neuropsychopharmacology* 16(5): 366–75.

Chambers, C.D., Hernandez-Diaz, S., Van Marter, L.J., *et al.* (2006) Selective serotonin-reuptake inhibitors and risk of persistent pulmonary hypertension of the newborn. *New England Journal of Medicine* 354(6): 579–87.

Chambers, H. (2006a) General Principles of anti-microbial therapy, pp.1095–1110. In: Brunton, L., Lazo, J., Parker, K. (eds) *Goodman & Gilman's: The Pharmacological Basis of Therapeutics*, 11th edition. McGraw-Hill: New York.

Chambers, H. (2006b) Protein synthesis inhibitors and miscellaneous antibacterial agents, pp.1173–202. In: Brunton, L., Lazo, J., Parker, K. (eds) *Goodman & Gilman's: The Pharmacological Basis of Therapeutics*, 11th edition. McGraw-Hill: New York.

Chan, L. (2002) Drug-nutrient interaction in clinical nutrition. *Current Opinion in Clinical Nutrition and Metabolic Care* 5(3): 327–32.

Chappell, B. (1993) Implications of switching antiepileptic drugs. *Prescriber* 4(18): 37–8.

Clerk, N., Emery, S. (2002) Epilepsy in Pregnancy, pp. 386–402. In: Jordan, S. (ed.) *Pharmacology for Midwives: the Evidence Base for Safe Practice*. Palgrave Macmillan: Basingstoke.

Cockshott, W.P., Thompson, G.T., Howlett, L., Seeley, E. (1982) Intramuscular or intralipomatous injections? *New England Journal of Medicine* 307(6): 356–8.

Committee of Public Accounts (2006) *A Safer Place for Patients: Learning to Improve Patient Safety*. Committee of Public Accounts, House of Commons: The Stationery Office: London.

Cooper, C.B., Tashkin, D.P. (2005) Recent development in inhaled therapy in stable chronic obstructive pulmonary disease. *British Medical Journal* 330: 640–4.

Courtenay, M., Butler, M. (2000) *Nurse Prescribing: Principles and Practice*. Greenwich Medical Media: London.

Cunningham Owens, D.G. (1999) *A Guide to the Extrapyramidal Side-Effects of Antipsychotic Drugs*. Cambridge University Press: Cambridge.

Currier, G., Simpson, G. (2001) Risperidone liquid concentrate and oral lorazepam versus intramuscular haloperidol and intramuscular lorazepam for treatment of psychotic patients. *Journal of Clinical Psychiatry* 62(3): 153–7.

Dahlof, B., Sever, P.S., Poulter, N.R., *et al.* ASCOT Investigators. (2005) Prevention of cardiovascular events with an antihypertensive regimen of amlodipine adding perindopril as required versus atenolol adding bendroflumethiazide as required, in the Anglo-Scandinavian Cardiac Outcomes Trial-Blood Pressure Lowering Arm (ASCOT-BPLA): a multicentre randomised controlled trial. *Lancet* 366(9489): 895–906.

Darwish, M., Kirby, M., Robertson, P. Jr., Hellriegel, E., Jiang, J.G. (2006) Comparison of equivalent doses of fentanyl buccal tablets and arteriovenous differences in fentanyl pharmacokinetics. *Clinical Pharmacokinetics* 45(8): 843–50.

Davis, S. (2006) Insulin, oral hypoglycaemic agents, and the pharmacology of the endocrine pancreas, pp.1613–45. In: Brunton, L., Lazo, J., Parker, K. (eds) *Goodman and Gilman's: The Pharmacological Basis of Therapeutics*, 11th edition. McGraw-Hill: New York.

DCCTRG (Diabetes Control and Complications Trial Research Group) (2001) Influence of intensive diabetes treatment on body weight and composition of adults with type 1 diabetes in the Diabetes Control and Complications Trial. *Diabetes Care* 24(10): 1711–21.

Degner, D., Grohmann, R., Kropp, S., *et al.* (2004) Severe adverse drug reactions of antidepressants: results of the German multicenter drug surveillance program AMSP. *Pharmacopsychiatry* 37(Suppl.1): S39–45.

Department of Health (DH) (2000) *An Organisation with a Memory*. Report of an expert group on learning from adverse events in the NHS. The Stationery Office: London.

Department of Health (DH) (2006) *Immunisation against Infectious Disease: the Green Book*. The Stationery Office: London. http: //www.dh.gov.uk/en/Policyandguidance/Healthandsocialcaretopics/Greenbook/DH_4097254 accessed May 2007

Doran, C. (2003) *Prescribing Mental Health Medication*. Routledge: London.

Dougherty, L. (2004) Drug administration: cytotoxic drugs, pp. 228–56. In: Dougherty, L. and Lister, S. (eds) *The Royal Marsden Hospital Manual of Clinical Nursing Procedures*, 6th edition. Blackwell Science: Oxford.

Dresser, G., Spence, D., Bailey, D. (2000) Pharmacokinetic-pharmacodynamic consequences and clinical relevance of cytochrome P450 3A4 inhibition. *Clinical Pharmacokinetics* 38(1): 41–57.

Dresser, G., Bailey, D., Leake, B., *et al.* (2002) Fruit juices inhibit organic anion transporting polypeptide-mediated drug uptake to decrease the oral availability of fexofenadine. *Clinical Pharmacology and Therapeutics* 71(1): 11–20.

Dubus, J., Marguet, C., Le Roux, P., Brouard, J., Huiart, L. (2001) Local side-effects of inhaled corticosteroids in asthmatic children. *Allergy* 56(10): 944–9.

Edwards, I.R., Aronson, J.K. (2000) Adverse drug reactions: definitions, diagnosis, and management. *Lancet* 356: 1255–9.

El Menyar, A.A. (2006) Drug-induced myocardial infarction secondary to coronary artery spasm in teenagers and young adults. *Journal of Postgraduate Medicine* 52(1): 51–6.

Endrenyi, L. (2007) Pharmacokinetics: principles and clinical applications, pp. 50–61. In: Kalant, H., Grant, D., Mitchell, J. (eds) *Principles of Medical Pharmacology*, 7th edition. Saunders, Elsevier: Toronto.

Engeland, A., Haldorsen, T., Andersen, A., Tretli, S. (1996) The impact of smoking habits on lung cancer risk: 28 years' observation of 26,000 Norwegian men and women. *Cancer Causes and Control* 7: 366–76.

Fairgrieve, S., Jackson, M., Jonas, P., *et al.* (2000) Population based, prospective study of the care of women with epilepsy in pregnancy. *British Medical Journal* 321: 674–5.

Farwell, A., Braverman, L. (2006) Thyroid and anti-thyroid drugs, pp.1511–72. In: Brunton, L., Lazo, J., Parker, K. (eds) *Goodman and Gilman's: The Pharmacological Basis of Therapeutics*, 11th edition. McGraw-Hill: New York.

Fonzo-Christe, C., Vukasovic, C., Wasilewski-Rasca, A.F., Bonnabry, P. (2005) Subcutaneous administration of drugs in the elderly: survey of practice and systematic literature review. *Palliative Medicine* 19(3): 208–19.

193

Food and Drug Administration, Health and Human Services (2007) Laxative drug products for over-the-counter human use; psyllium ingredients in granular dosage forms. Final rule. *Federal Register* 72(60): 14669–74.

French, D.D., Campbell, R., Spehar, A., Cunningham, F., Foulis, P. (2005) Outpatient medications and hip fractures in the US. *Drugs and Aging* 22(10): 877–85.

Frier, B., Fisher, B. (2002) Diabetes Mellitus, pp. 641–82. In: Haslett, C., Chilvers, E., Boon, N., Colledge, N. (eds) *Davidson's Principles & Practice of Medicine*. Churchill Livingstone: Edinburgh.

Fugh-Berman, A. (2000) Herb-drug interactions. *Lancet* 355: 9198; 134–8.

Garrett, A., Fitzgerald, M. (2004) Coxibs and cardiovascular disease. *New England Journal of Medicine* 351: 1709–11.

Genuth, S., Alberti, K.G., Bennett, P., *et al*. Expert Committee on the Diagnosis and Classification of Diabetes Mellitus (2003) Follow-up report on the diagnosis of diabetes mellitus. *Diabetes Care* 26: 3160–7.

Ginsberg, G., Hattis, D., Sonawane, B., *et al*. (2002) Evaluation of child/adult pharmacokinetic differences from a database derived from the therapeutic drug literature. *Toxicological Sciences* 66(2): 185–200.

Ginsberg, G., Hattis, D., Russ, A., Sonawane, B. (2005) Pharmacokinetic and pharmacodynamic factors that can affect sensitivity to neurotoxic sequelae in elderly individuals. *Environmental Health Perspectives* 113(9): 1243–9.

Gitlin, M., Altshuler, L.L., Frye, M.A., *et al*. (2004) Peripheral thyroid hormones and response to selective serotonin reuptake inhibitors. *Journal of Psychiatry and Neuroscience* 29(5): 383–6.

Gladstone, J. (1995) Drug administration errors: a study into the factors underlying the occurrence and reporting of drug errors in a district general hospital. *Journal of Advanced Nursing* 22(4): 628–37.

Glinoer, D., Abalovich, M. (2007) Unresolved questions in managing hypothyroidism during pregnancy. *British Medical Journal* 335: 300–2.

Gooch, K., Culleton, B.F., Manns, B.J., *et al*. (2007) NSAID use and progression of chronic kidney disease. *American Journal of Medicine* 120(3): 280.e1–7.

Greenway, K. (2004) Using the ventrogluteal site for intramuscular injection. *Nursing Standard* 18(25): 39–42.

Griffiths, T.H., Jordan, S. (2002) Corticosteroids: implications for nursing practice. *Nursing Standard* 17(12): 43–54.

Grossman, E., Messerli, F. (2006) Long-term safety of antihypertensive therapy. *Progress in Cardiovascular Disease* 49(1): 16–25.

Gutstein, H., Akil, H. (2006) Opioid analgesics, pp. 547–90. In: Brunton, L., Lazo, J., Parker, K. (eds) *Goodman & Gilman's: The Pharmacological Basis of Therapeutics*, 11th edition. McGraw-Hill: New York.

Guy, W. (1976) *ECDEU Assessment Manual for Psychopharmacology*. US Dept. of Health, Education & Welfare: Washington DC.

Guyton, A.C., Hall, J.E. (2000) *Textbook of Medical Physiology*, 9th edition. W.B. Saunders: Kidlington.

Haddad, P.M., Wieck, A. (2004) Antipsychotic-induced hyperprolactinaemia: mechanisms, clinical features and management. *Drugs* 64(20): 2291–314.

Hancox, R., Aldridge, R., Cowan, J., *et al*. (1999) Tolerance to beta-agonists during acute bronchoconstriction. *European Respiratory Journal* 14: 283–7.

Hansen, D., Lou, H., Olsen, J. (2000) Serious life events and congenital malformations: a national study with complete follow-up. *Lancet* 356: 875–80.

Harada, K., Tsuruoka, S., Fujimura, A. (2001) Shoulder stiffness: a common adverse effect of HMG-CoA reductase inhibitors in women. *Internal Medicine* 40(8): 817–18.

REFERENCES

Hardy, B., Jordan, S. (2002) Drugs prescribed for mental illness, pp. 346–62. In: Jordan, S. (ed.) *Pharmacology for Midwives: the Evidence Base for Safe Practice*. Palgrave Macmillan: Basingstoke.

Hayes, D., Hendler, C.B., Tscheschlog, B., *et al.* (eds) (2003) *Medication Administration Made Incredibly Easy*. Springhouse, Lippincott Williams and Wilkins: Philadelphia.

Healy, D. (2004) *Psychiatric Drugs Explained*. Mosby: London.

Hendeles, L., Colice, G., Meyer, R. (2007) Withdrawal of albuterol inhalers containing chlorofluorocarbon propellants. *New England Journal of Medicine* 356: 1334–51.

Hendrick, V., Fukuchi, A., Altshuler, L., Widawski, M., Wertheimer, A., Brunhuber, M.V. (2001) Use of sertraline, paroxetine and fluvoxamine by nursing women. *British Journal of Psychiatry* 179: 163–6.

Hickson, M., D'Souza, A.L., Muthu, N., *et al.* (2007) Use of probiotic Lactobacillus preparation to prevent diarrhoea associated with antibiotics: randomised double blind placebo controlled trial. *British Medical Journal* 335: 80–3.

Hirsch, I. (2005) Insulin analogues. *New England Journal of Medicine* 352(2): 174–83.

Holmer Pettersson, P., Jakobsson, J., Owall, A. (2006) Plasma concentrations following repeated rectal or intravenous administration of paracetamol after heart surgery. *Acta Anaesthesiologica Scandinavia* 50(6): 673–7.

Hoogerwerf, W., Pasricha, P. (2006) Pharmacotherapy of gastric acidity, pp. 967–81. In: Brunton, L., Lazo, J., Parke, K. (eds) *Goodman & Gilman's: The Pharmacological Basis of Therapeutics.*, 11th edition. McGraw-Hill: New York.

Howard, L. (2001) Enteral and parenteral nutrition therapy, pp. 470–90. In: Braunwald, E., Fauci, A., Kasper, D., Hauser, S., Longo, D., Jameson, J. (eds) *Harrison's Principles of Internal Medicine*, 15th edition. McGraw-Hill: New York.

Hu, X.H., Bull, S.A., Hunkeler, E.M., *et al.* (2004) Incidence and duration of side effects and those rated as bothersome with selective serotonin reuptake inhibitor treatment for depression: patient report versus physician estimate. *Journal of Clinical Psychiatry* 65(7): 959–65.

Hurria, A., Lichtman, S. (2007) Pharmacokinetics of chemotherapy in the older patient. *Cancer Control* 14(1): 32–43.

International Conference on Harmonisation (ICH) (1996) *ICH Harmonised Tripartite Guideline for Good Clinical Practice*. Institute of Clinical Research: Marlow, Buckinghamshire.

Irl, C., Hasford, J. (2000) Assessing the safety of drugs in pregnancy: the role of prospective cohort studies. *Drug Safety* 22: 169–77.

Jackson, E. (2006a) Diuretics, pp. 737–70. In: Brunton, L., Lazo, J., Parker, K. (eds) *Goodman & Gilman's: The Pharmacological Basis of Therapeutics,* 11th edition. McGraw-Hill: New York.

Jackson, E. (2006b) Renin and angiotensin, pp. 789–821. In: Brunton, L., Lazo, J., Parker, K. (eds) *Goodman & Gilman's: The Pharmacological Basis of Therapeutics,* 11th edition. McGraw-Hill: New York.

Jehle, P., Micheler, C., Jehle, D., Breitig, D., Boehm, B. (1999) Inadequate suspension of neutral protamine Hagendorn (NPH) insulin in pens. *Lancet* 354: 1604–7.

Jevon, P., Ewens, B. (2002) *Monitoring the Critically Ill Patient*. Blackwell Science: Oxford.

Joint Specialty Committee on Renal Medicine of the Royal College of Physicians of London and the Renal Association (JSC) (2006) *Chronic Kidney Disease in Adults: UK Guidelines for Identification, Management and Referral*. Royal College of Physicians: London.

Jordan, S. (2002a) Managing adverse drug reactions: an orphan task. Developing nurse-administered evaluation checklists. *Journal of Advanced Nursing* 38(5): 437–8.

Jordan, S. (2002b) *Pharmacology for Midwives: the Evidence Base for Safe Practice.* Palgrave: Basingstoke.

Jordan, S. (2006) Infant feeding and analgesia in labour: the evidence is accumulating. *International Breastfeeding Journal* 1(1): 25. doi: 10.1186/1746–4358–1-25 tp: //www.internationalbreastfeedingjournal.com/content/1/1/25 (accessed 8 Jan 2007).

Jordan, S. (2007) Adverse drug reactions: reducing the burden of treatment. *Nursing Standard* 21(34): 35–41.

Jordan, S., White, J. (2001) Non-steroidal anti-inflammatory drugs: implications for nursing practice. *Nursing Standard* 15(23): 45–52.

Jordan, S., Griffiths, H., Griffith, R. (2003) Continuing professional development: administration of medicines. Part 2 Pharmacology. *Nursing Standard* 18(3): 45–55.

Jordan, S., Knight, J., Pointon, D. (2004) Monitoring Adverse Drug Reactions: Scales, Profiles and Checklists. *International Nursing Review* 51: 208–21.

Jordan, S., Emery, S., Bradshaw, C., Watkins, A., Friswell, W. (2005) The impact of intrapartum analgesia on infant feeding. *British Journal of Obstetrics and Gynaecology* 112: 927–34.

Kahn, S.E., Haffner, S.M., Heise, M.A., *et al.* (2006) ADOPT Study Group. Glycemic durability of rosiglitazone, metformin, or glyburide monotherapy. *New England Journal of Medicine* 355(23): 2427–43. Erratum in: *N Engl J Med* (2007); 356(13): 1387–8.

Kaklamanos, M., Perros, P. (2007) Milk alkali syndrome without the milk. *British Medical Journal* 335: 397–8.

Kane, J.M. (ed.) (1999) *Managing the Side Effects of Drug Therapy in Schizophrenia.* Science Press: London.

Karch, A. (2006) *Focus on Nursing Pharmacology*, 3rd edition. Lippincott: Philadelphia.

Katz, P. (2003) Optimizing medical therapy for gastroesophageal reflux disease. *Reviews in Gastroenterological Disorders* 3(2): 59–69.

Katzung, B., Julius, D. (2001) Histamine, serotonin and the ergot alkaloids, pp. 265–91. In: Katzung, B. (ed.) *Basic and Clinical Pharmacology*, 8th edition. McGraw-Hill: New York.

Keeley, D. (1993) How to achieve better outcome in treatment of asthma in general practice. *British Medical Journal* 307: 1261–3.

Kelly, J. (2000) *Adverse Drug Effects: A Nursing Concern.* Whurr Publishers: London.

Klaassen, C.D. (2001) Principles of toxicology and treatment of poisoning, pp. 67–80. In: Hardman, J., *et al.* (eds) *Goodman & Gilman's: The Pharmacological Basis of Therapeutics*, 10th edition. McGraw-Hill: New York.

Koh, T.W. (2001) Risk of torsades de pointes from oral erythromycin with concomitant carbimazole (methimazole) administration. *Pacing and Clinical Electrophysiology* 24(10): 1575–6.

Koren, G. (2001) Special Aspects of perinatal and pediatric pharmacology, pp.1025–35. In: Katzung, B. (ed.) *Basic and Clinical Pharmacology*, 8th edition. McGraw Hill: New York.

Koren, G., Pastuszak, A., Ito, S. (1998) Drugs in pregnancy. *New England Journal of Medicine* 338(16): 1128–37.

Korytkowski, M., Bell, D., Jacobsen, C., Suwannasari, R. for the FlexPen Study Team (2003) A multicenter, randomized open-label, comparative, two-period crossover trial of preference, efficacy and safety profile of a prefilled disposable pen and conventional vial/syringe for insulin injections in patients with type 1 or 2 diabetes mellitus. *Clinical Therapeutics* 25: 2836–48.

Lattimore, K., Donn, S., Kaciroti, N., Kemper, A., Neal, C., Vazquez, D. (2005) Selective serotonin reuptake inhibitor (SSRI) use during pregnancy and effects on the fetus and neonate. *Journal of Perinatology* 25: 595–604.

REFERENCES

Le Souëf, P. (1999) Asthma in children. *Medicine* 27(9): 54–8.

Lee, W., Senior, J. (2005) Recognizing drug-induced liver injury. *Toxicologic Pathology* 33: 155–64.

Lemmer, B. (2003) Rhythms in therapeutics of cardiovascular disease, pp.192–209. In: Redfern, P. (ed.) *Chronotherapeutics*. Pharmaceutical Press: London.

Levey, A., Bosch, J., Lewis, J., Greene, T., Rogers, N., Roth, D. (1999) A more accurate method to estimate glomerular filtration rate from serum creatinine: a new prediction equation. *Annals of Internal Medicine* 130: 461–70.

Lipworth, B.J., Wilson, A.M. (2002) Dose response to inhaled corticosteroids: benefits and risks. (Abstracts of quality assessed systematic reviews). In: The Cochrane Library, Issue 3, Oxford. Update Software.

Lutomski, D., Bottorff, M., Sangha, K. (1995) Pharmacokinetic optimisation of the treatment of embolic disorders. *Clinical Pharmacokinetics* 28(1): 67–92.

Macfarlane, A., Gissler, M., Bolumnar, F., Rasmussen, S. (2003) The availability of perinatal health indicators in Europe. *European Journal of Obstetrics and Gynecology and Reproductive Biology* 111: S15–32.

Majerus, P., Tollefsen, D. (2006) Drugs acting on the blood and blood forming organs, pp.1433–88. In: Brunton, L., Lazo, J., Parker, K. (eds) *Goodman & Gilman's: The Pharmacological Basis of Therapeutics,* 11th edition. McGraw-Hill: New York.

Markowitz, G., Perazella, M. (2005) Drug-induced renal failure: a focus on tubulointerstitial disease. *Clinica Chimica Acta* 351: 31–47.

Maxwell, C.J., Hogan, D.B., Campbell, N.R.C., Ebly, E.M. (2000) Nifedipine and mortality risk in the elderly: relevance of drug formulation, dose and duration. *Pharmacoepidemiological Drug Safety* 9: 11–23.

McCowen, K.C., Garber, J.R., Spark, R. (1997) Elevated serum thyrotropin in thyroxine-treated patients with hypothyroidism given sertraline. *New England Journal of Medicine* 337(14): 1010–11.

McElhatton, P., Bateman, D., Evans, C., Pughs, K., Thomas, S. (1999) Congential anomalies after prenatal ecstasy exposure. *Lancet* 354: 1441–2.

McKenry, L., Salerno, E. (2003) *Pharmacology in Nursing*, 21st edition. Mosby: St Louis.

McNamara, J. (2006) Pharmacotherapy of the epilepsies, pp. 501–25. In: Brunton, L., Lazo, J., Parker, K. (eds) *Goodman & Gilman's: The Pharmacological Basis of Therapeutics,* 11th edition. McGraw-Hill: New York.

Meyer, F., Troger, U., Rohl, F. (1996) Adverse non-drug reactions: an update. *Clinical Pharmacology and Therapeutics* 60: 347–52.

Michel, T. (2006) Treatment of myocardial ischaemia, pp. 823–44. In: Brunton, L., Lazo, J., Parker, K. (eds) *Goodman & Gilman's: The Pharmacological Basis of Therapeutics,* 11th edition. McGraw-Hill: New York.

Micheletto, C., Guerriero, M., Tognella, S., Dal Negro, RW. (2005) Effects of HFA- and CFC-beclomethasone dipropionate on the bronchial response to methacholine (MCh) in mild asthma. *Respiratory Medicine* 99(7): 850–5.

Millar, J. (2001) Consultations owing to adverse drug reactions in a single practice. *British Journal of General Practice* 51: 130–1.

Milman, N., Bergholt, T., Byg, K.E., Eriksen, L., Hvas, A.M. (2007) Reference intervals for haematological variables during normal pregnancy and postpartum in 434 healthy Danish women. *European Journal of Haematology* 79(1): 39–46.

Morrell, M.J. (2003) Reproductive and metabolic disorders in women with epilepsy. *Epilepsia* 44(Suppl 4): 11–20.

Nabulsi, M., Tamim, H., Sabra, R., *et al.* (2005) Equal antipyretic effectiveness of oral and rectal acetaminophen: a randomized controlled trial. *BioMed Central Pediatrics* 6(5): 35.

Naysmith, M., Nicholson, J. (1998) Nasogastric drug administration. *Professional Nurse* 13(7): 424–51.

Neugut, A., Ghatak, A., Miller, R. (2001) Anaphylaxis in the United States: an investigation into its epidemiology. *Archives of Internal Medicine* 161(1): 15–21.

NICE (2002) *Management of Type 2 Diabetes: Management of Blood Glucose.* NICE: London.

NICE (2004a) *Chronic Obstructive Pulmonary Disease: Management of Chronic Obstructive Pulmonary Disease in Adults in Primary and Secondary Care.* Clinical Guideline 12. NICE: London.

NICE (2004b) *Depression: Management of Depression in Primary and Secondary Care.* Clinical Guideline 23. NICE: London.

NICE (2004c) *The Epilepsies: Diagnosis and Management of the Epilepsies in Adults in Primary and Secondary Care.* Clinical Guideline 20. NICE: London.

NICE (2004d) *Type 1 Diabetes: Diagnosis and Management of Type 1 Diabetes in Children, Young People and Adults.* Clinical Guideline 15. NICE: London.

NICE (2006a) *Management of Hypertension in Adults in Primary Care.* Clinical Guideline 34. NICE: London.

NICE (2006b) *Bipolar disorder: management of bipolar disorder in adults, children and adolescents in primary and secondary care.* Clinical guideline 38. NICE: London.

NICE (2006c) *Inhaled Insulin for the Treatment of Diabetes (Types 1 and 2).* Technology Appraisal 113. NICE: London.

Nisbet, A. (2006) Intramuscular gluteal injections in the increasingly obese population. *British Medical Journal* 332: 637–8.

Nisbet, J., Sturtevant, J., Prins, J. (2004) Metformin and serious adverse effects. *Medical Journal of Australia* 180(2): 53–4.

O'Keane, V., March, M. (2007) Depression in pregnancy. *British Medical Journal* 334: 1003–5.

Oiknine, R., Mooradian, A.D. (2003) Drug therapy of diabetes in the elderly. *Biomedical Pharmacotherapeutics* 57(5–6): 231–9.

Pasricha, P. (2006) Treatment of disorders of bowel motility and water flux, pp. 983–1008. In: Brunton, L., Lazo, J., Parker, K. (eds) *Goodman & Gilman's: The Pharmacological Basis of Therapeutics*, 11th edition. McGraw-Hill: New York.

Pea, F., Furlanut, M. (2001) Pharmacokinetic aspects of treating infections in the intensive care unit: focus on drug interactions. *Clinical Pharmacokinetics* 40(11): 833–68.

Perahia, D.G., Kajdasz, D.K., Desaiah, D., Haddad, P.M. (2005) Symptoms following abrupt discontinuation of duloxetine treatment in patients with major depressive disorder. *Journal of Affective Disorders* 89(1–3): 207–12.

Perrone, R., Madias, N., Levey, A. (1992) Serum creatinine as an index of renal function: new insights into old concepts. *Clinical Chemistry* 38(10): 1933–53.

Perucca, E., Berlowitz, D., Birnbaum, A., *et al.* (2006) Pharmacological and clinical aspects of antiepileptic drug use in the elderly. *Epilepsy Research* 68(Suppl 1): S49–63.

Petri, W. (2006) Penicillins, cephalosporins and other beta-lactam antibiotics, pp.1127–54. In: Brunton, L., Lazo, J., Parker, K. (eds) *Goodman & Gilman's: The Pharmacological Basis of Therapeutics*, 11th edition. McGraw-Hill: New York.

Picchioni, M., Murray, R. (2007) Schizophrenia. *British Medical Journal* 335: 91–5.

Pirmohamed, M., James, S., Meakin, S., *et al.* (2004) Adverse drug reactions as cause of admission to hospital: prospective analysis of 18820 patients. *British Medical Journal* 329: 15–19.

Poirier, M., Olivero, O., Walker, D., Walker, V. (2004) Perinatal genotoxicity and carcino-genicity of anti-retroviral nucleoside analog drugs. *Toxicology and Applied Pharmacology* 199: 151–61.

Poole-Wilson, P.A., Lubsen, J., Kirwan, B.A., *et al.* A coronary disease trial investigating outcome with nifedipine gastrointestinal therapeutic system investigators (2004)

REFERENCES

Effect of long-acting nifedipine on mortality and cardiovascular morbidity in patients with stable angina requiring treatment (ACTION trial): randomised controlled trial. *Lancet* 364(9437): 849–57.

Pratt, R.J., Pellowe, C.M., Wilson, J.A., *et al*. (2007) epic2: National evidence-based guidelines for preventing healthcare-associated infections in NHS hospitals in England. *Journal of Hospital Infection* 65(Suppl 1): S1–64.

Preston, S., Hegadoren, K. (2004) Glass contamination in parenterally administered medication. *Journal of Advanced Nursing* 48(3): 266–70.

Railton, D. (2007) *Knowledge Set: Medication*. Harcourt Education, Heinemann: Oxford.

Rang, H., Dale, M., Ritter, J., Flower, R. (2007) *Pharmacology*, 6th edition. Churchill Livingstone, Elsevier: Edinburgh.

Royal College of General Practitioners (RCGP) (1985) *What Sort of Doctor? Assessing Quality of Care in General Practice*. Report from General Practice no.23. Royal College of General Practitioners: London.

RCP (Royal College of Psychiatrists and the British Psychological Society) (2003) *Schizophrenia: Full National Clinical Guideline on Core Interventions in Primary and Secondary Care*. Royal College of Psychiatrists and the British Psychological Society: London.

RCP/BHS (2006) *Management of Hypertension in Adults in Primary Care*. Royal College of Physicians: London.

Redmond, A., McCelland, H. (2006) Chronic kidney disease: risk factors, assessment and nursing care. *Nursing Standard* 21(10): 48–55.

Rodrigo, E., de Francisco, A.L., Escallada, R., *et al*. (2002) Measurement of renal function in pre-ESRD patients. *Kidney International* 61: S11–S17.

Roger, M., King, L. (2000) Drawing up and administering intramuscular injections: a review of the literature. *Journal of Advanced Nursing* 31(3): 574–82.

Ross, S., Solters, D. (1995) Heparin and haematoma: does ice make a difference? *Journal of Advanced Nursing* 21: 434–9.

Routledge, P. (2004) Adverse drug reactions and interactions, pp. 91–127. In: Talbot, J., Walker, P. (eds) *Stephens' Detection of New Adverse Drug Reactions*. Wiley: Chichester.

Ruggiero, R. (2006) Visible embryo pharmaceutical guide to drugs in pregnancy. http: // www.visembryo.com/baby/pharmaceuticals.html (accessed February 2007).

Russell, A.R., Murch, S.H. (2006) Could peripartum antibiotics have delayed health consequences for the infants? *British Journal of Obstetrics and Gynaecology* 113: 758–65.

Salpeter, S., Buckley, N., Ormiston, T., Salpeter, E. (2006) Meta-analysis: effect of long-acting ß-agonists on severe asthma exacerbations and asthma-related deaths. *Annals of Internal Medicine* 144(12): 904–12.

Sampson, H.A., Munoz-Furlong, A., Bock, S.A., *et al*. (2005) Symposium on the definition and management of anaphylaxis: summary report. J*ournal of Allergy and Clinical Immunology* 115(3): 584–91.

Sampson, H.A., Muñoz-Furlong, A., Campbell, R.L., *et al*. (2006) Symposium on the definition and management of anaphylaxis: summary report. *Journal of Allergy and Clinical Immunology* 117: 391–7.

Sazawal, S., Hiremath, G., Dhingra, U., Malik, P., Deb, S., Black, R.E. (2006) Efficacy of probiotics in prevention of acute diarrhoea: a meta-analysis of masked, randomised, placebo-controlled trials. *Lancet Infectious Diseases* 6(6): 374–82.

Schenk, B.E., Kuipers, E.J., Klinkenberg-Knol, E.C., *et al*. (1999) Atrophic gastritis during long-term omeprazole therapy affects serum vitamin B12 levels. *Alimentary Pharmacology and Therapeutics* 13(10): 1343–6.

Schimmer, B., Parker, K. (2006) Adrenocorticotropic hormone; adrenocortical steroids and their synthetic analogues, pp. 1587–1612. In: Brunton, L., Lazo, J., Parker, K. (eds) *Goodman & Gilman's: The Pharmacological Basis of Therapeutics*, 11th edition. McGraw-Hill: New York.

REFERENCES

Schmidt, L., Dalhoff, K. (2002) Food-drug interactions. *Drugs* 62(10): 1481–502.

Sharma, A., Pischon, T., Hardt, S., Kunz, I., Luft, F. (2001) Beta-adrenergic receptor blockers and weight gain: a systematic analysis. *Hypertension* 37: 250–4.

Shear, H. (2007) Adverse Drug Reactions, pp. 803–11. In: Kalant, H., Grant, D., Mitchell, J. (eds) *Principles of Medical Pharmacology,* 7th edition. Saunders, Elsevier: Toronto.

Shin, H., Kim, M. (2006) Subcutaneous tissue thickness in children with type I diabetes. *Journal of Advanced Nursing* 54(1): 29–34.

Sholter, D., Armstrong, P. (2000) Adverse effects of corticosteroids on the cardiovascular system. *Canadian Journal of Cardiology* 16(4): 505–11.

Skorecki, K., Green, J., Brenner, B. (2001) Chronic renal failure, pp.1551–62. In: Braunwald, E., Fauci, A., Kasper, D., *et al.* (eds) *Harrison's Principles of Internal Medicine*, 15th edition. McGraw-Hill: New York.

Slordal, L., Spigset, O. (2006) Heart failure induced by non-cardiac drugs. *Drug Safety* 29(7): 567–86.

Smith, S., Duell, D., Martin, B. (2008) *Clinical Nursing Skills: Basic to Advanced Skills*, 7th edition. Pearson, Prentice Hall: New Jersey.

Snodin, D.J. (2004) Toxicology and adverse drug reactions, pp.128–66. In: Talbot, J., Walker, P. (eds) *Stephens' Detection of New Adverse Drug Reactions*. Wiley: Chichester.

Solensky, R., Earl, H., Gruchalla, R. (2002) Lack of penicillin resensitization in patients with a history of penicillin allergy after receiving repeated penicillin courses. *Archives of Internal Medicine* 162: 822–6.

Stern, R., Chosidow, O., Wintroub, B. (2001) Cutaneous drug reactions, pp. 336–42. In: *Harrison's Principles of Internal Medicine*, 15th edition. McGraw-Hill: New York.

Stevens, L., Levey, A. (2005) Chronic kidney disease in the elderly – how to assess risk. *New England Journal of Medicine* 352(20): 2122–4.

Strachan, M., Ewing, F., Frier, B., McCrimmon, R., Deary, I. (2003) Effects of acute hypoglycaemia on auditory information processing in adults with Type 1 Diabetes. *Diabetologia* 46: 97–105.

Suntharalingam, G., Perry, M., Ward, S., *et al.* (2006) Cytokine storm in a phase 1 trial of the anti-CD28 monoclonal antibody TGN1412. *New England Journal of Medicine* 355: 1018–28.

Talbot, J., Stephens, M.D.B. (2004) Clinical trials: collection of safety data and establishing the adverse drug reaction profile, pp.167–242. In: Talbot, J., Walker, P. (eds) *Stephens' Detection of New Adverse Drug Reactions*. Wiley: Chichester.

Taylor, D., Paton, C., Kerwin, R. (2005) *The South London and Maudsley NHS Trust 2005–6 Prescribing Guidelines*. Taylor & Francis: London.

Thomson, F., Naysmith, M., Lindsay, A. (2000) Managing drug therapy in patients receiving enteral and parenteral nutrition. *Hospital Pharmacist* 7(6): 155–64.

Tierney, W. (2003) Adverse outpatient drug events – a problem and opportunity. *New England Journal of Medicine* 348(16): 1587–9.

UKPDS Group (UK Prospective Diabetes Study Group) (1998) Intensive blood-glucose control with sulphonylureas or insulin compared with conventional treatment and risk of complications in patients with type 2 diabetes (UKPDS 33). *Lancet* 352(9131): 837–53. Erratum in: *Lancet* 1999 Aug 14; 354(9178): 602.

Vesalainen, R., Ekholm, E., Jartii, T., Tahvanainen, K., Kaila, T., Erkkola, R. (1999) Effects of tocolytic treatment with ritodrine on cardiovascular autonomic regulation. *British Journal of Obstetrics and Gynaecology* 106: 238–43.

Viramontes, B.E., Camilleri, M., McKinzie, S., Pardi, D.S., Burton, D., Thomforde, G.M. (2001) Gender-related differences in slowing colonic transit by a 5-HT3 antagonist in subjects with diarrhea-predominant irritable bowel syndrome. *American Journal of Gastroenterology* 96: 2671–6.

van Walraven, C., Mamdani, M.M., Wells, P.S., Williams, J.I. (2001) Inhibition of serotonin reuptake by antidepressants and upper gastrointestinal bleeding in elderly patients: retrospective cohort study. *British Medical Journal* 323(7314): 655–8.

Wald, A. (2007) Fecal incontinence in adults. *New England Journal of Medicine* 356(16): 1648–55.

Walker, M. (2005) Status epilepticus: an evidence based guide. *British Medical Journal* 331: 673–7.

Wallace, A.W., Amsden, G.W. (2002) Is it really OK to take this with food? *Journal of Clinical Pharmacology* 42(4): 437–43.

Warfarin Antiplatelet Vascular Evaluation Trial Investigators (2007) Oral anticoagulant and antiplatelet therapy and peripheral arterial disease. *New England Journal of Medicine* 357(3): 217–27.

Weingart, S., Gandhi, T., Seger, A., *et al.* (2005) Patient reported medication symptoms in primary care. *Archives of Internal Medicine* 165: 234–40.

Whitaker, R. (2004) The case against antipsychotic drugs: a 50-year record of doing more harm than good. *Medical Hypotheses* 62: 5–13.

White, M., Sander, N. (1999) Asthma from the perspective of the patient. *Journal of Allergy and Clinical Immunology* 104;2(Part 2): 47–52.

WHO (2005) *Hospital Care for Children. Guidelines for the management of common illnesses with limited resources.* WHO: Geneva.

Wigham, C., Hodson, S. (1987) Physiological changes in the cornea of the ageing eye. *Eye* 1: 190–6.

Wilkinson, G. (2001) Pharmacokinetics, pp. 3–30. In: Hardman, J., Limbard, L., Molinoff, P., Ruddon, R., Goodman Gilman, A. (eds) *Goodman & Gilman's: The Pharmacological Basis of Therapeutics*, 10th edition. McGraw-Hill: New York.

Williams, B., Poulter, N., Brown, MJ., *et al.* (2004) British Hypertension Society Guidelines: Guidelines for management of hypertension: report of the fourth working party of the British Hypertension Society. *Journal of Human Hypertension* 18: 139–85.

Wilson, A.M., Dempsey, O.J., Coutie, W.J., Sims, E.J., Lipworth, B.J. (1999) Importance of drug-device interaction in determining systemic effects of inhaled corticosteroids. *Lancet* 353(9170): 2128.

Wood, A.J. (2001) Adverse reactions to drugs, pp. 430–8. In: Braunwald, E., Fauci, A., Kasper, D., Hauser, S., Longo, D., Jameson, J. (eds) *Harrison's Principles of Internal Medicine*, 15th edition. McGraw-Hill: New York.

Workman, B. (2000) Safe injection technique. *Nursing Standard* 13(39): 47–53.

Wright, D. (2002) Medication Administration in Nursing Homes. *Nursing Standard* 16(42): 33–8.

Yoshida, K., Smith, B., Kumar, R. (1999) Psychotropic drugs in mothers' milk: a comprehensive review of assay methods, pharmacokinetics and of safety of breast feeding. *Journal of Psychopharmacology* 13(1): 64–80.

Young, J.B., Dunlap, M.E., Pfeffer, M.A., *et al.* Candesartan in Heart Failure Assessment of Reduction in Mortality and Morbidity (CHARM) Investigators and Committees. (2004) Mortality and morbidity reduction with Candesartan in patients with chronic heart failure and left ventricular systolic dysfunction: results of the CHARM low-left ventricular ejection fraction trials. *Circulation* 110(17): 2618–26.

Yusuf, S., Sleight, P., Pogue, J., Bosch, J., Davies, R., Dagenais, G. (2000) Effects of an angiotensin-converting-enzyme inhibitor, ramipril, on cardiovascular events in high-risk patients. The Heart Outcomes Prevention Evaluation Study Investigators. *New England Journal of Medicine* 342(3): 145–53.

Zillich, A., Garg, J., Basu, S., Bakris, G., Carter, B. (2006) Thiazide diuretics, potassium and the development of diabetes. *Hypertension* 48: 219–24.

Bibliography/Further Reading

Galbraith, A., Bullock, S., Manias, E., Hunt, B., Richards, A. (2007) *Fundamentals of Pharmacology*, 2nd edition. Addison Wesley: Harlow.

Griffith, R., Griffiths, H., Jordan, S. (2003) Continuing professional development: administration of medicines. Part 1; the law. *Nursing Standard* 18(2): 47–54.

Jordan, S., Griffiths, H., Griffith, R. (2003) Continuing professional development: administration of medicines. Part 2; pharmacology. *Nursing Standard* 18(3): 45–54.

Herfindal, E., Gourley, D. (eds) (2000) *Textbook of Therapeutics and Disease Management*, 7th edition. Lippincott: Philadelphia.

Index

Locators shown in *italics* refer to boxes, figures and tables.

203

INDEX